Imen Ouertani

Climate change and infectious animal diseases

Imen Ouertani

Climate change and infectious animal diseases

ScienciaScripts

Imprint

Cover image: www.ingimage.com

This book is a translation from the original published under ISBN 978-620-6-72901-3.

Publisher:
Sciencia Scripts
is a trademark of
Dodo Books Indian Ocean Ltd. and OmniScriptum S.R.L publishing group

120 High Road, East Finchley, London, N2 9ED, United Kingdom
Str. Armeneasca 28/1, office 1, Chisinau MD-2012, Republic of Moldova, Europe
Managing Directors: Ieva Konstantinova, Victoria Ursu
info@omniscriptum.com

Printed at: see last page
ISBN: 978-620-8-36781-7

Table of contents

Introduction

Climate change refers to long-term variations in temperature and weather patterns. These can be natural variations, due for example to those of the solar cycle or to massive volcanic eruptions. However, since the 1800s, human activities have been the main cause of climate change, mainly due to the burning of fossil fuels such as coal, oil and gas. Emissions that cause climate change come from all regions of the planet and affect everyone, but some countries produce more than others. The seven biggest emitters of greenhouse gases are China, the United States, India, the European Union, Indonesia, the Russian Federation and Brazil, and in 2020 they were responsible for half of all emissions. (Badillo 2024).

The impact of climate change on the emergence and re-emergence of animal diseases has been confirmed by a majority of OIE Member Countries and Territories, according to a global survey conducted by the OIE among all its National Delegates and presented by Dr Peter Black, Australian Rapporteur, at the Assembly. The three emerging diseases most frequently cited by 126 of the 174 OIE Member States that took part in the study are: bluetongue, Rift Valley fever and West Nile fever. In addition, 58% of them identified the recent appearance of at least one emerging or re-emerging disease in their territory as being directly linked to climate change. Climate change is altering the nature and likelihood of animal disease outbreaks in a given region. Under its influence, it has been observed, for example, that epizootics due to vector-borne diseases have become more frequent, and now affect a wider geographical area. However, health risks still vary from one region to another (Black and Nunn 2009, French Ministry of Agriculture 2023).

Disease emergence is driven by multiple factors, including environmental change (including climate change), social and demographic change (including globalization), and changes to public health policies and systems. The same factors can favor the re-emergence of endemic diseases (i.e., increased incidence or re-emergence in the form of epidemics). Climate and climate change can have direct effects on the emergence and re-emergence of infectious diseases by influencing the survival of pathogens, the survival and reproduction of arthropod vectors, water contamination and, in the case of zoonoses, the abundance of reservoir hosts (i.e. microbe-carrying animals) (Ogden and Gachon 2019).

Early detection is the key to rapid diagnosis and response, and to effective management of emerging animal diseases. Some emerging animal diseases are contagious, spreading rapidly and regardless of borders. Rapid response and management of animal disease at an early stage are essential for the implementation of effective biosecurity measures, the objectives of which are :

- Limit the spread of the disease to other farms and prevent an epidemic, or limit its consequences;

- Implement appropriate control measures and communicate them effectively;

- Reduce the cost, difficulty and scale of control, and achieve better results. The consequences of disease or epidemics can be reduced if hazards are detected early and information is rapidly exchanged between the partners involved. A well-functioning breeder-veterinarian-authority network in the field, with optimal transmission of information, is of crucial importance in the fight against emerging animal diseases (Barnouin and VOURC'H 2004).

These diseases can have significant consequences in terms of public and animal health, as well as in economic and social terms. Through their socio-economic impact, they closely concern the primary animal production sector, in particular livestock farmers (Diricks 2018).

Part 1: Overview of climate change and emerging diseases

A. Climate change

I. Definitions

1. The climate

The term "climate" is defined by the World Meteorological Organization (WMO) as the "synthesis of weather conditions in a given region, characterized by the long-term statistics of variables in the state of the atmosphere". Seasonal changes, such as the transition from winter to spring, summer and autumn in temperate zones, and from humidity to drought in tropical regions, are also part of climate (MelloukiHanane 2023).

2. Climate change

The term "climate change" refers to variations in temperature and weather conditions over the long term. These variations may be a natural phenomenon, but since the beginning of the 19th century they have mainly resulted from human activity, notably the use of fossil fuels (such as coal, oil and gas), which produce greenhouse gases (United Nations 2024).

3. Greenhouse effect

The greenhouse effect is a natural phenomenon, resulting from the presence in the atmosphere of gases (water vapour, carbon dioxide, methane, etc.) that absorb the thermal infrared radiation emitted by the earth's surfaces, without which the average global temperature would be around -18°C instead of +15°. This heat reserve helps maintain temperatures that are conducive to life on Earth (Seguin and Soussana 2008).

II. Main manifestations of climate change

Many people think that climate change is mainly about higher temperatures. But rising temperatures are only the beginning of the problem. As the Earth is an interconnected system, a change in one place can have repercussions everywhere else.

Currently, the consequences of climate change include intense droughts, water shortages, severe fires, rising sea levels, flooding, melting polar ice, catastrophic storms and declining biodiversity (Barnouin and Sache 2010, Ogden and Gachon 2019, United Nations 2024).

1. Temperature rise

One of the main manifestations of climate change is the rise in the earth's surface temperature. Global surface temperature is 1.1°C higher than in the 1800s (fig.1), before the industrial revolution. The last decade (2011-2020) was the warmest on record, and each of the preceding decades was warmer than any decade since 1850. In almost all regions of the world, very hot days and heat waves are on the increase. The year 2020 was one of the hottest on record. Rising temperatures are causing an increase in heat-related illnesses, and can make work and travel more difficult. In addition, forest fires start more easily and spread faster when temperatures are higher. (Barnouin and Sache 2010, United Nations 2024).

In a series of United Nations reports, thousands of scientists and government assessors agreed that containing the global temperature rise to within 1.5°C would help prevent the most severe climate impacts and maintain a livable climate. Yet, on the basis of current national climate plans, the central estimate of warming is expected to reach 2.7°C by the end of the century, compared with pre-industrial levels, but there is a 10% chance of warming reaching 3.5°C. A global temperature rise in excess of 5°C cannot be ruled out (fig.2) (Quiggin, De Meyer et al. 2021, United Nations 2024).

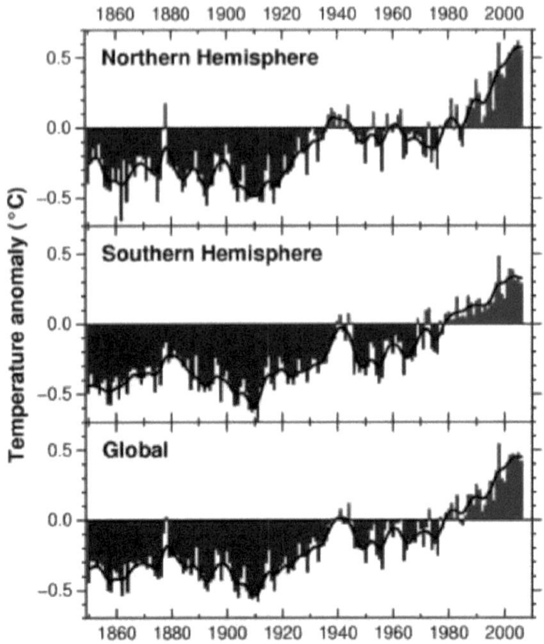

Figure 1: Hemispheric and global surface temperature trends
(Barnouin and Sache 2010)

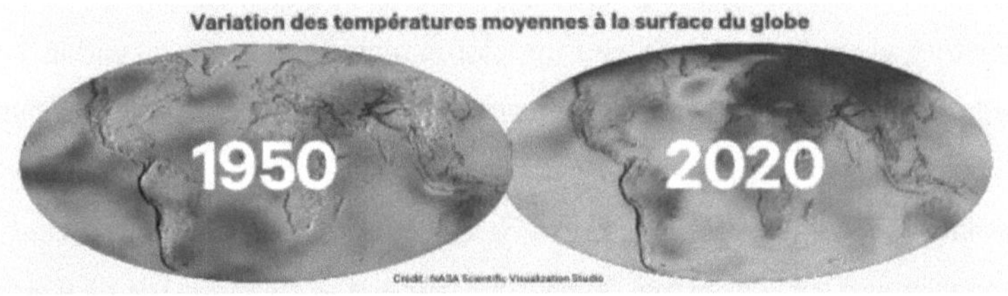

Figure 2: Variation in global average surface temperatures
(Quiggin, De Meyer et al. 2021)

Over time, rising temperatures are disrupting climatic conditions and upsetting the usual natural balance. This situation poses numerous risks for human beings and all other forms of life on Earth. Biological indicators, such as movements of animal populations on land and at sea, and changes in the dates of seasonal agricultural activities, also point to the onset of global warming. Although difficult to quantify, these elements are important and have consequences in many areas of professional activity, where they are widely taken into account (Puget, Blanchet et al. 2010, United Nations 2024).

2. Increased severity of storms

Changes in temperature in turn lead to changes in precipitation. This translates into more violent and frequent storms, which can cause flooding and landslides, destroy homes and communities, and cost billions of dollars (Barnouin and Sache 2010, United Nations 2024).

3. Increased drought

More and more regions are facing water shortages. Droughts can trigger destructive sand and dust storms, moving billions of tons of sand across continents. With desertification, arable land is also shrinking. Today, many people are at risk of running out of water. In the Sahel, in 2020, some 13.4 million people in Mali, Niger and Burkina Faso were reported to be in need of humanitarian aid due to drought. Compared with the historical benchmark, the global area of land affected by drought doubled in 2019. The lack of water during the 2012 US drought was forecast to reduce GDP growth by 0.5 to 1 percentage point, with natural disasters declared in 71% of counties. In 2020, drought in China's Yunnan province affected 1.5 million people. Around 100 rivers were cut off, 180 reservoirs dried up and 140 irrigation wells were no longer supplied with sufficient water (Puget, Blanchet et al. 2010, Quiggin, De Meyer et al. 2021, United Nations 2024).

By 2040, North Africa, the Middle East, Western and Central Europe and Central America will see more than 10% of their respective populations affected by severe and prolonged drought (fig 3).

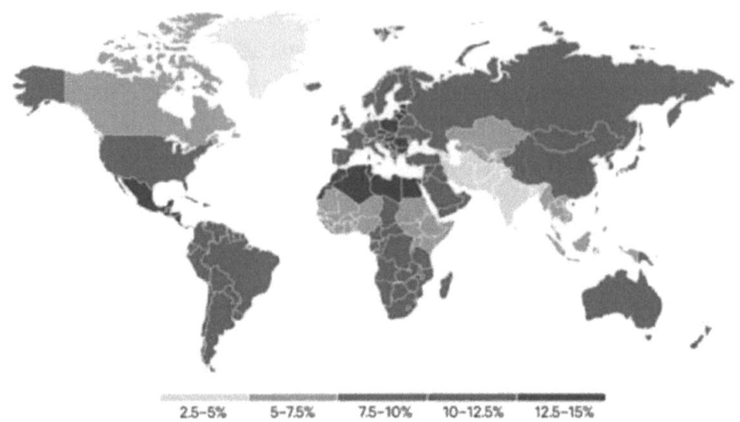

Figure 3: Proportion of the population experiencing severe and prolonged drought each year

(Quiggin, De Meyer et al. 2021)

4. Global warming and rising oceans

The oceans are absorbing much of the heat generated by global warming. This is causing ice caps to melt and sea levels to rise, threatening coastal and island communities. Coastal flooding is likely to occur over a longer period. The central long-term estimate of sea level rise is around 12 meters, if temperature increases are maintained at 2°C. This rise could occur over 500 or 10,000 years: the timescales are extremely uncertain (fig.4).

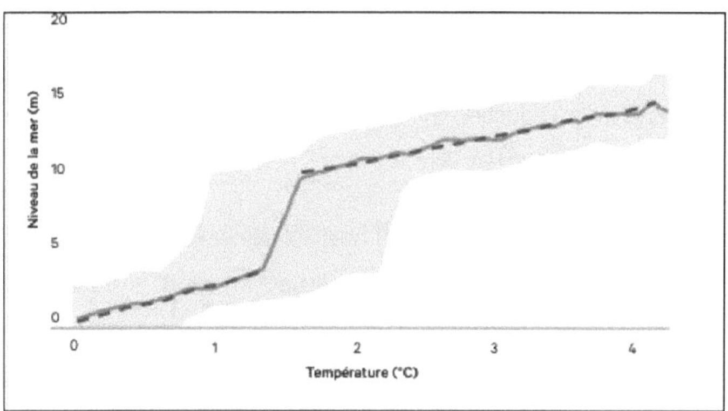

Figure 4: Sea level rise as a function of long-term global temperature increase

(Quiggin, De Meyer et al. 2021)

Oceans also absorb carbon dioxide from the atmosphere. As carbon dioxide increases, the ocean becomes more acidic, endangering marine life. One billion people now live on land less than 10 meters above current high tide lines, including 230 million at less than one meter. In 2020, there were 23% more floods than the annual average of 163 events over the period 2000-2019, and 18% more flood-related deaths than the annual average of 5,233 (Barnouin and Sache 2010, Puget, Blanchet et al. 2010, Quiggin, De Meyer et al. 2021, United Nations 2024).

5. Loss of biodiversity

Climate change is threatening the survival of species on land and in the oceans. The higher the temperatures, the greater the risks. Forest fires, extreme weather conditions, pest species and disease are just some of the many threats posed by climate change. While some species are able to move and survive, others cannot (Barnouin and Sache 2010, United Nations 2024).

6. Food shortage

The rise in hunger and malnutrition around the world is largely due to climate change and the increase in extreme weather events. Fish stocks, crops and livestock are at risk of destruction or loss of productivity. In addition, heat stress can lead to a reduction in water resources and grassland for grazing (Puget, Blanchet et al. 2010).

In recent years, drought and regional heat waves have caused crop losses of 20-50% worldwide. In Australia, severe drought caused a 50% collapse in wheat harvests for two consecutive years (2006-2007) and 50% crop failure. In Central and Northern Europe, the 2018 heatwave resulted in multiple crop failures and yield losses of up to 50%. In China's Liaoning province, years of drought have led to a 20-25% reduction in corn harvests. By 2040, the proportion of the world's cropland affected by severe drought, equivalent to that experienced in Central Europe in 2018 (yield reductions of 50%), is likely to reach 32% each year, more than three times the historical average (Quiggin, De Meyer et al. 2021, United Nations 2024).

7. Increased health risks

Changing weather conditions favor the spread of diseases such as malaria. Extreme weather events lead to an increase in illness and death, and put a strain on health systems. Other health risks include increased famine and malnutrition in regions where it is impossible to grow or find enough food (Barnouin and Sache 2010, United Nations 2024).

Climate change is responsible for changes in vector distribution and abundance. They impact the dynamics of pathogen transmission and spread, and contribute to the evolution of new pathogen characteristics such as virulence and antimicrobial resistance. They are also responsible for modifying the migratory trajectories of birds (Tazerji, Nardini et al. 2022).

8. Poverty and displacement

Climate change accentuates the factors that contribute to poverty. For example, floods can sweep away slums, destroying homes and livelihoods; heat can make outdoor work difficult. Every year, weather-related disasters displace 23 million people, making them even more vulnerable to poverty (Barnouin and Sache 2010, Masson-Delmotte, Zhai et al. 2021, United Nations 2024).

III. Factors behind climate change

Climate variations, whether natural or unnatural, are caused by a number of factors. Initially, it will be simpler to consider only so-called natural variations (Barnouin and Sache 2010).

1. Natural factors in climate change

The Earth's climate varies naturally, without human intervention, according to cycles and punctual events. Global climate variability is normal, and is due to fluctuations in ocean currents, volcanic eruptions, solar radiation, astronomical parameters and other components of the climate system. These changes remain small and have few consequences (Barnouin and Sache 2010, Swynghedauw and Wemeau 2021).

2. Man's role in global warming

It's important to distinguish between global warming and climate change, warming being one of the causes of climate change.

When greenhouse gas emissions multiply, these gases act like a blanket around the Earth, trapping the sun's heat. This is a natural phenomenon that helps maintain average temperatures. However, with the increasing concentration of greenhouse gases in the atmosphere as a result of human activity, it is intensifying, leading to global warming and climate change. Today, the Earth is warming faster than ever (United Nations 2024).

Scientists have shown that human activity is responsible for a very large proportion of global warming over the last 200 years. Human activities, producing emissions mainly of carbon dioxide (CO_2), methane (CH_4) and nitrous oxide (N_2O), are at the root of climate change. These emissions result, for example, from the use of fuel to power vehicles or coal to heat buildings. Clearing land and forests can also release carbon dioxide. Agriculture and combustion engines are major sources of methane emissions. Excessive use of nitrogen fertilizers and certain chemical processes are responsible for the emission of nitrous oxide (N_2O) (Fig 5).

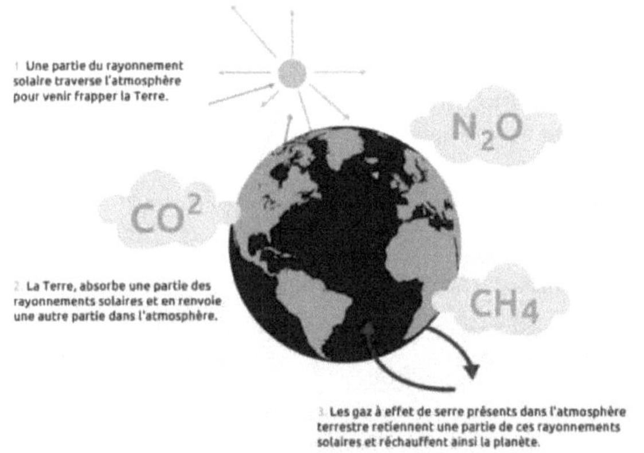

Figure 5: Greenhouse gases responsible for global warming

(Badillo 2024)

The energy, industry, transport and construction sectors, as well as land use, are among the main emitters of greenhouse gases (Gérin, Gosselin et al. 2003, Masson-Delmotte, Zhai et al. 2021, United Nations 2024).

The great forest massifs of the tropics (Amazon Basin, Congo Basin, Indonesia and New Guinea) play a fundamental role in terms of climate. However, these forest areas are subject to intense human pressure, in particular deforestation for timber sales or oil palm cultivation. The climatic consequences of deforestation are reflected locally in desertification, which leads to soil drying

(Barnouin and Sache 2010).

A number of other human actions play a part in climate change, such as pollution of terrestrial waters by industrial wastewater, the intensification of livestock farming and food production, and the excessive and uncontrolled use of pesticides (Gérin, Gosselin et al. 2003, Masson-Delmotte, Zhai et al. 2021).

The FAO report entitled The Shadow of Livestock Farming concludes that the livestock sector is largely responsible for environmental damage at all levels, from local to global. The report considers that livestock production must be at the heart of policies on climate change, soil degradation, water scarcity, water pollution and biodiversity loss. Clearly, there is a wide range of possible responses that can be implemented at production sector, country or regional level. The general trend towards intensive, industrial livestock farming is set to continue, as human societies seek to improve yields and reduce the land required for livestock production. The same arguments of profitability and reduction of available land apply to aquaculture (Black and Nunn 2009, FAO 2020).

B. Emerging and re-emerging infectious animal diseases

I. Definitions

1. Infectious disease

Infectious diseases are caused by pathogens (bacteria, viruses, parasites and fungi) and spread, directly or indirectly, from one person to another.

These diseases can be divided into three categories: those with a high mortality rate, those causing significant disability in the population and those which, given the rapidity and unpredictability of their spread, can have serious consequences on a global scale (WHO).

There are two modes of transmission for infectious diseases: direct and indirect. Indirect transmission involves a vector. Vector-borne diseases are best described as a "pathogenic complex". This complex is made up of the three major elements of the epidemiological cycle: the pathogen, the host and the vector, and the relationships between them (Chevalier, Courtin et al. 2015, Shongo, Lubala et al. 2020).

2. Pathogen

These are living beings (organisms belonging to one of the 4 following families: bacteria, viruses, parasites, microscopic fungi) or inanimate beings (toxins), said to be pathogenic because they are likely to cause infections or toxi-infections (Ajana et al 2022).

3. Triggering factors

Causes or risks associated with the presence of emerging or re-emerging diseases, such as anthropogenic, environmental, behavioral, demographic or biological factors (Tazerji, Nardini et al. 2022).

4. Emerging disease

Emergence, in its event-based dimension, corresponds to the occurrence of an unexpected situation involving an element of the unknown as well as "proximity to oneself". The event-related value attached to the notion of an emerging disease can lead to the presentation of any significant health problem, especially if it occurs in epidemic form, as one of emergence. In epidemiological terms, emergence can lead to a high level of media coverage and the adoption of draconian measures based on the precautionary principle (e.g. BSE, H5N1 and H N1 influenza) (Barnouin and Sache 2010).

The World Health Organization (WHO) defines emerging diseases as: "Emerging diseases are those which appear in a population for the first time, or which probably existed previously and experience a sudden increase in incidence or geographical distribution" (WHO 2024).

The World Organisation for Animal Health (OIE) defines Emerging Diseases as a new appearance, in an animal, of a disease, infection or infestation with significant repercussions on animal or human health (SARS, avian influenza, for example) (Wang, Thitithanyanont et al. 2021, Wannous 2024).

Another more detailed definition "An emerging animal disease is an animal disease whose incidence (i.e. the number of new cases of diseased animals) increases significantly in a given region, in a given population (animal or human), and over a given period of time, this being independent of the disease's usual seasonal fluctuations." (Toma and Thiry 2003, Diricks 2018).

A definition shared by WHO and WHOA defines an emerging disease as: "An emerging disease is a disease whose actual incidence increases significantly in a given population, in a given region and during a given period, compared with the usual epidemiological situation for that disease. This definition applies equally to human, animal and plant diseases. Although emerging diseases are mainly infectious in nature, they may also involve other types of disease, whether toxic, metabolic or other" (Shongo, Lubala et al. 2020).

An emerging disease can follow four dynamics of evolution over time, depending on the number of cases recorded (fig. 6)

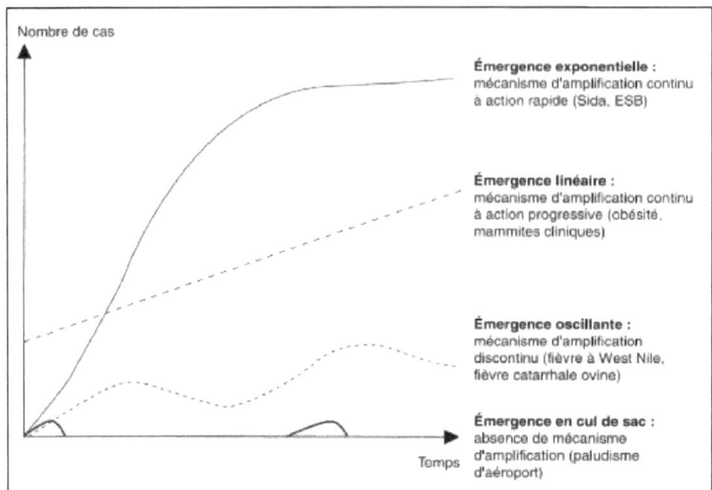

Figure 6: Temporal dynamics of the number of cases and type of emerging disease

(Barnouin and Sache 2010)

Several descriptions can be attributed to emerging diseases: (Diricks 2018)

- It may be a new disease caused by a previously unknown pathogen, such as Schmallenberg disease, which until 2011 was an unknown disease until it was identified following a series of abortions.

- It may be a disease caused by a mutated micro-organism, such as avian flu.

- It may be a disease that exists in a given region, but whose number of new cases in animals increases over a given period, e.g. tick-borne diseases such as ehrlichiosis, babesiosis and borreliosis, which will follow the seasonal increase in ticks or as a result of climate change.

- there are animal diseases at risk of emergence. These are diseases that are not yet present in a given region but exist in other countries or regions, and for which the risk of introduction is real, e.g. the risk of introduction of foot-and-mouth disease from neighboring countries (Diricks 2018).

5. Re-emerging disease

WHO defines a re-emerging disease as "a disease that at one time represented a major health problem before declining and then reappearing recently, causing major health complications (e.g. plague, yellow fever) (Wang, Thitithanyanont et al. 2021, Wannous 2024).

These are diseases that have existed in a given region, have been eradicated or have disappeared, but are reappearing or are at risk of reappearing in that region, e.g. Belgium was heavily contaminated with bovine brucellosis until the late 1980s, before becoming "officially free" in 2003. Between 2010 and 2013, several outbreaks of brucellosis were again identified in Belgium (Diricks 2018).

II. Conditions for disease emergence

Three conditions must be met for a contagious animal disease to emerge in a region and cause an epidemic/pandemic (fig. 7):

1. it must be introduced into a farm with animals susceptible to the disease (for example, through the introduction of a sick animal following trade from an infected country) and infect the animals;

2. it must become established (persist) on the farm and in the region (for example, because of the survival of insect vectors as a result of global warming);

3. it must spread among neighboring farms, for example, as a result of the movement of insect vectors, and possibly throughout the region, for example, as a result of the transport of infected animals. This takes more or less time, depending on the degree of contagiousness of the diseases (Diricks 2018).

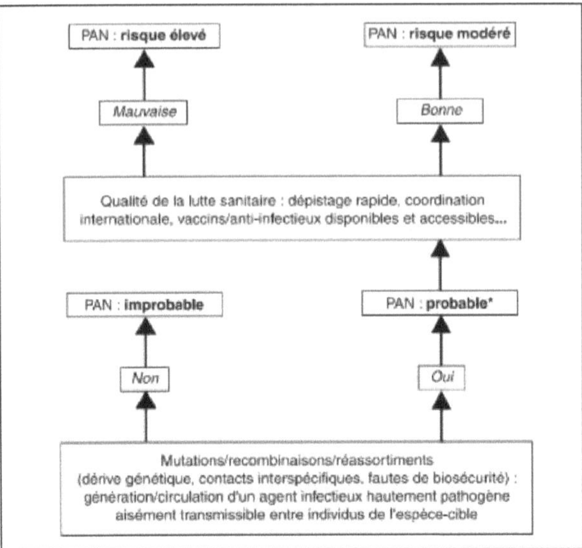

Figure 7: Conditions for the emergence of a Pandemic-Panzootic Disease (PAN)

(Barnouin and Sache 2010)

III. the determinants of the emergence of an infectious disease :

The determinants of disease emergence are multiple: they may include factors linked to the evolution of pathogens, human and animal demographics and changes in farming practices, and environmental changes (fig. 8). Social and cultural factors, such as eating habits and religious beliefs, also play a role (Dufour 2017, WHO 2024).

The average rise in temperature, even in winter, allows insects to persist, transmitting animal diseases in unusual regions. The number of mosquitoes and ticks capable of transmitting numerous diseases is on the rise. Examples are the facilitated survival of Culicoides, vectors of the blue tongue disease virus, in winter and the increase in tick numbers in Northern Europe (Diricks 2018).

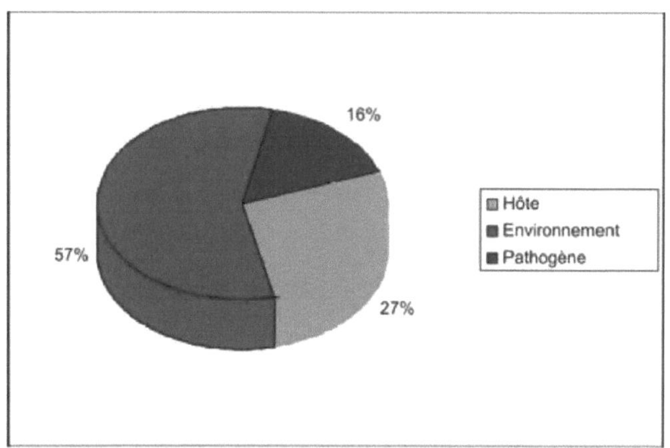

Figure 8: Relative weight (in percent) of the three determinants of infectious disease emergence

(Pepin, Boireau et al. 2007)

1. Pathogen-related factors :

Infectious pathogens evolve like all living species. However, their evolution is generally rapid, given their short life cycle and mode of reproduction. Whether viruses or bacteria, their multiplication depends on their interactions with the species they infect. The greater the number of interactions, the greater the multiplication of pathogens, and the greater the evolution of these pathogens. RNA viruses (especially segmented RNA viruses such as influenza viruses) are prime candidates for such evolution. The inevitable transcription errors can lead to evolutionary modifications. The multiplicity of viruses in the same family is also a factor in the exchange of genetic material between them, which can lead to adaptive evolutions. In recent years, several diseases have emerged as a result of these genetic evolutions.

Recent worrying increases in multi-resistant bacteria are another example of the harmful evolution of pathogens.

Consequently, the changes in pathogens responsible for the emergence of infectious diseases are essentially linked to genome modification (Pepin, Boireau et al. 2007):

- The acquisition of virulence or antibiotic resistance genes, such as the increase in toxinogenicity of *Clostridium* strains that have emerged in certain countries;

- Loss of avirulence gene(s) (well described in the world of plant-parasitic nematodes and for certain bacterial diseases);

- Gene rearrangement at the origin of "superbugs" like the 1918 Spanish flu virus.

The collective fight against major animal diseases has also contributed to the creation of healthy but immunologically naïve populations, i.e. perfectly receptive to the pathogens eradicated from these countries. The genetic selection applied to certain animal productions, by improving production, has not contributed significantly to the robustness of individuals against major diseases. For example, foot-and-mouth disease, which is still commonplace and relatively benign in many southern countries, poses a major threat to improved, disease-free livestock in northern countries (Dufour 2017).

2. Factors linked to human activity :

Human activity is certainly responsible for the emergence or re-emergence of many infectious or parasitic diseases, through a number of factors:

- The globalization of trade in people, animals and their products is a particularly important factor in the rapid and massive spread of pathogens. Moreover, it is extremely difficult to combat this spread effectively, given the sheer volume of movements involved, and the impossibility of checking the health status of people before they travel, particularly in the case of mass population movements due to conflict, for example. In addition, very short transport times encourage the movement of individuals in the incubation phase. For animals, controls (serological tests and quarantines) are theoretically possible, but are not always carried out. Last but not least, wild animals (migratory birds in particular) escape any possibility of control. Recent episodes of avian influenza in livestock illustrate these risks of pathogen circulation and regular introductions through wildlife movements (Dufour 2017).

- The increase in human population densities in various parts of the planet (Asia in particular) has led to a correlative increase in animal densities to feed these populations. These densities favor the emergence of new pathogens and their circulation, all the more so as in these often still-developing zones, the relationships between domestic animals and human populations are very close (Dufour 2017).

- Changes in people's behavior can also lead to the emergence of certain diseases. For example, the growing popularity of outdoor activities over the last 30 years has encouraged contact with certain vectors that are potential carriers of disease. The return to nature also applies to animals in developed countries, whose confinement in open-air livestock farms is increasingly frowned upon by consumers in these countries (development of open-air poultry and pig farms). This "free-range" practice thus leads to new risks of re-emergence through contact with wild fauna carrying infections often eradicated from farms at great expense (bovine tuberculosis, Aujeszky's disease, for example) (Dufour 2017).

Finally, technological changes linked to progress have, sometimes insidiously (development of *Hsteria* in relation to the development of the cold chain), and other times more explosively (bovine spongiform encephalopathy in relation to changes in meat and bone meal manufacturing), been the cause of the emergence of major diseases (Dufour 2017).

- The recent craze for NACs (new pets) also presents risks of disease emergence or re-emergence. Remember that American prairie dogs can carry *Yersinia pestis,* that reptiles silently harbor infrequent salmonella serotypes in their intestines, and that rabies has at least once been reintroduced to France by an Egyptian dogfish (Dufour 2017).

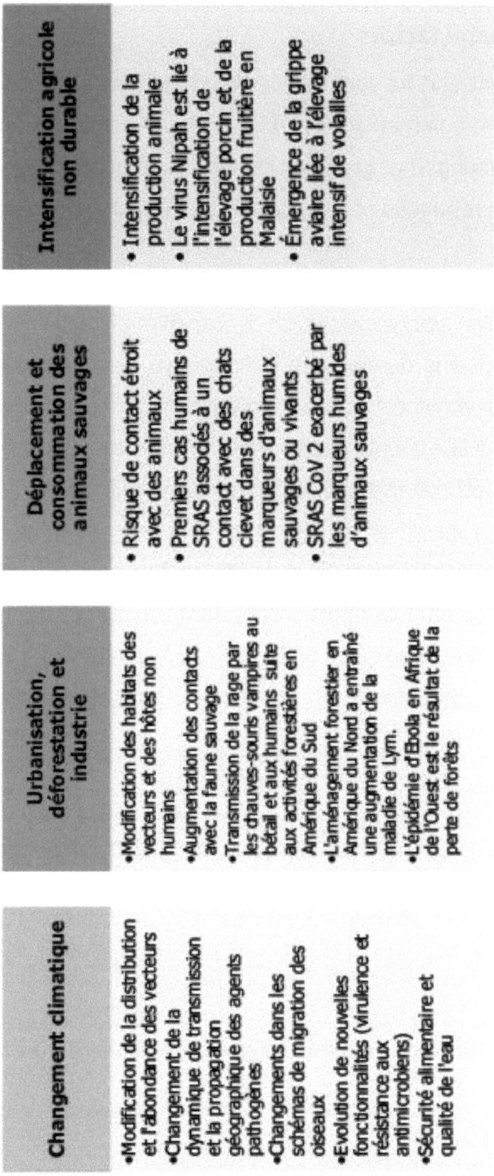

Changement climatique	Urbanisation, déforestation et industrie	Déplacement et consommation des animaux sauvages	Intensification agricole non durable
•Modification de la distribution et l'abondance des vecteurs •Changement de la dynamique de transmission et la propagation géographique des agents pathogènes •Changements dans les schémas de migration des oiseaux •Evolution de nouvelles fonctionnalités (virulence et résistance aux antimicrobiens) •Sécurité alimentaire et qualité de l'eau	•Modification des habitats des vecteurs et des hôtes non humains •Augmentation des contacts avec la faune sauvage •Transmission de la rage par les chauves-souris vampires au bétail et aux humains suite aux activités forestières en Amérique du Sud •L'aménagement forestier en Amérique du Nord a entraîné une augmentation de la maladie de Lym. •L'épidémie d'Ebola en Afrique de l'Ouest est le résultat de la perte de forêts	• Risque de contact étroit avec des animaux • Premiers cas humains de SRAS associés à un contact avec des chats cievet dans des marqueurs d'animaux sauvages ou vivants • SRAS CoV 2 exacerbé par les marqueurs humides d'animaux sauvages	• Intensification de la production animale • Le virus Nipah est lié à l'intensification de l'élevage porcin et de la production fruitière en Malaisie • Émergence de la grippe aviaire liée à l'élevage intensif de volailles

Figure 9: The main factors in the emergence of infectious diseases linked to human activities

3. Environmental factors

The environment and its spontaneous modifications also play a role in the emergence or re-emergence of certain diseases. First and foremost, global warming is altering the geographical distribution and densities of flying vectors and the reservoirs of apterous vectors (small rodents and their ticks).

Global warming is certainly responsible for the establishment in southern France *of Aedes albopictus*, which is capable of transmitting numerous arboviroses, including dengue and chikungunya. Another striking feature of the changing environment is the significant increase in the number of wild animals over the last twenty years. These animals are infected with a variety of pathogens (for example, wild boar carry the Aujeszky's disease virus, or ibex in the Bargy massif are infected with *Brucella melitensis*, or badgers are infected with *Mycobacterium bovis* in the south-west). These animals were probably initial victims of infections by farm animals, but now that these infections have been eradicated on farms, infected wild fauna constitute a risk of re-emergence, particularly for 'free-range" farms (Dufour 2017).

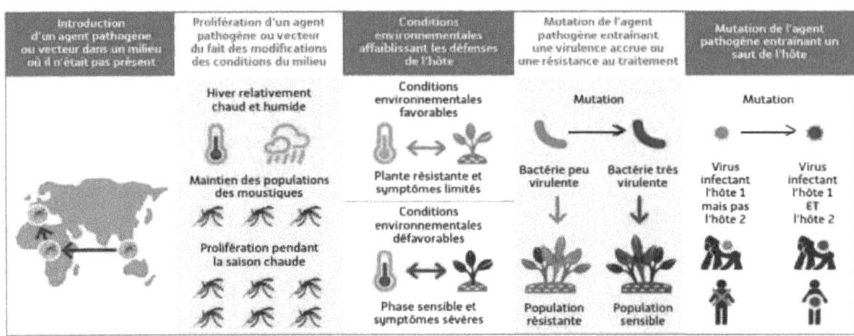

Figure 10: Factors likely to generate emerging diseases

(Sanguine 2021)

Part 2: Climate change and emerging and re-emerging infectious animal diseases

Local contextual parameters, such as the epidemiological situation of animal populations (domestic and wild), farming methods and pre-existing risk management systems, on the one hand, and climate change on the other, influence the emergence or re-emergence of animal diseases. Today, the study of emerging diseases is mainly focused on terrestrial vertebrates, particularly domestic ones, due to better monitoring of their proximity to humans and the economic impact of their diseases (Thornton, Jones et al. 2010).

A. Impact of climate change

Climate change is bringing about major changes in animal physiology, in the regions in which they are present and in population movements, as well as in the epidemiological dynamics of animal diseases, particularly where vectors or reservoirs exist. It is, however, part of a multifactorial causality involving other factors such as the intensification of livestock farming and international trade, anthropogenic deforestation and soil artificialisation. Finally, animal populations are exposed to variable health risks on a global scale (French Ministry of Agriculture 2023).

I. Impact on animal physiology

Human and animal species have had to adapt to periods of glaciation and warming, drought and so on. These slow environmental changes have contributed to population migrations, and induced progressive genomic or epigenetic modifications in individuals, optimizing their adaptation to cold, heat or reduced water availability. Today's rapidly changing climate raises questions about the impact of climate change on the health of individuals and their adaptive capacities at different life stages and in different populations. Climate change can have a direct impact on animal physiology: droughts and heat waves cause heat stress, leading to suffering, dehydration, sometimes fatal cardio-respiratory disorders, and so on. These effects manifest themselves in weight loss, reproductive disorders and behavioral changes that, in the long term, threaten the general health of animal populations and can alter the productive yields of livestock (Ministry of Agriculture 2023).

Non-communicable diseases (metabolic or reproductive disorders) can thus be the direct consequence of weather conditions, themselves impacted by climate change. In the case of livestock, these effects can be exacerbated by the quantitative and qualitative alteration of animal feed during extreme weather events (drought, heatwaves, floods). Reduced forage yields, the lower nutritional value of cereals and pasture grass (lower concentrations of water-soluble carbohydrates and nitrogen; higher concentrations of lignin and cell wall components), difficulties in accessing water, etc., are all the less well tolerated by animals as their immune systems are affected, particularly during periods of high heat (Ministry of Agriculture 2023).

Climate change is also having an impact on the food intake of wild animals, which are finding it difficult to feed due to changes in plant cover or the disappearance of certain prey. As a result, they have to move outside their usual territory, even into areas occupied by domestic animals or humans. The resulting contacts can be the source of contamination (French Ministry of Agriculture 2023).

II. Impact on the modification of animal habitats

Climate change leads to the displacement of animal populations, modifying their habitats. Locally, species can settle in areas where they were previously considered exotic. The emergence of the zoonotic Nipah virus in the 1990s is correlated with the movement of bat populations into pig farming areas, which they contaminated. Anthropogenic destruction of living environments can also contribute to such mechanisms. Last but not least, changes in the routes or timing of seasonal animal migrations can sometimes increase the scale of epidemics, as in the case of avian influenza. Migratory birds are present in greater numbers, at the same time, at watering holes that act as staging posts on migration routes. The spread of influenza viruses can then be massive and rapid (French Ministry of Agriculture 2023).

Furthermore, the disturbances caused by warming can have repercussions on the health of migratory bird populations, but also of aquatic species: studies emphasize the speed of changes at work for fish and phytoplankton, likely to result in a shift (latitude and depth) and a reduction in the size of many fish species (Cheung, Sarmiento et al. 2013, Ministry of Agriculture 2023).

Sea ice is shrinking by around 13% per decade. It is the habitat, hunting ground and breeding ground of the polar bear, one of the most endangered mammal species. Farm animals are less able to protect themselves from rising temperatures. It is essential that animal welfare is taken into account (Swynghedauw and Wemeau 2021).

III. Impact on infectious diseases

The consequences of climate change on infectious diseases are better known than its diffuse effects on metabolic diseases. Increased temperatures can favor the spread of parasitic or vector-borne diseases and wild reservoir diseases, accelerate the biological development of certain pathogens and increase their populations, extend the range of insect vectors and therefore the incidence of associated diseases in regions previously little affected (Ministry of Agriculture 2023).

Some diseases are more likely to emerge as a result of geographical dispersal, via insects or wildlife, or as a result of trade in animals or animal products from infected countries.

Over the past 30 years, many infectious diseases have undergone a phase of emergence; Bovine spongiform encephalopathy (BSE) in Great Britain in 1986, West Nile virus infection in North America in 2000, highly pathogenic avian influenza H5N1 since 2003, Middle East *Respiratory Syndrom virus* (MERS-

CoV) in Saudi Arabia in 2012, Ebola virus fever which appeared in Africa (CAR) in 1962 and emerged particularly intensely and dramatically in 2014 in Guinea, then throughout West Africa. In 2017, in Southeast Asia, severe acute respiratory syndrome (SARS) in China in 2003. (Dufour 2017, Ogden and Gachon 2019).

In view of climate change, a 2005 report by the French Food Safety Agency (AFFSA) recommended the surveillance of six diseases in mainland France, 5 of which are vector-borne: Rift Valley fever, West Nile virus infection, canine leishmaniasis, leptospirosis, African horse sickness, bluetongue or ovine catarrhal fever (Afssa 2005, Swynghedauw and Wemeau 2021).

The processing and analysis of responses to a questionnaire carried out by WHOA in 2008, to assess how member countries might respond to the dual challenge of animal production and health, climate change and environmental change, addressed to all 172 WHOA Member Countries and Territories, showed that 58% of Members identified at least one emerging or re-emerging animal disease considered to be directly linked to climate change, and 30% identified at least one considered to be directly linked to environmental change. These responses enabled us to list the diseases most frequently cited as being associated with climate change or environmental change (Tab.1.) (Black and Nunn 2009).

Table I: List of animal diseases considered to be linked to climate change

(Black and Nunn 2009)

Maladies mentionnées au moins deux fois comme étant liées :	au changement climatique	au changement environnemental
Maladies vectorielles		
Fièvre catarrhale du mouton	✓	✓
Fièvre de la Vallée du Rift	✓	×
Fièvre à virus West Nile	✓	×
Peste équine	✓	×
Dermatose nodulaire contagieuse	✓	×
Leishmaniose	✓	✓
Maladie épizootique hémorragique	✓	×
Maladies transmises par des tiques	✓	✓
Maladies parasitaires (à l'exclusion de celles transmises par des tiques)	✓	✓
Pasteurellose	✓	×
Influenza aviaire	✓	✓
Fièvre charbonneuse	✓	✓
Charbon symptomatique	✓	×
Rage	✓	✓
Tuberculose	×	✓

1. Climate change and disease emergence due to the biological development of pathogens

Infectious diseases emerge due to changes in their geographical distribution and through "adaptive emergence", a genetic change affecting microorganisms that infect animals (usually wild animals) such that these microorganisms can infect humans and transmission may become possible between humans, in other words, a genetic adaptation that produces a new zoonotic disease. In some regions (Ogden and Gachon 2019).

Pathogens can now circulate in shorter timescales than the average disease incubation period. The increased circulation of pathogens increases the risk of contamination and the likelihood of new agents emerging from genetic combinations previously unimaginable (Angot 2009).

Thawing soils could also lead to the release of pathogens currently under control (anthrax bacteria or smallpox virus), or even unknown (survival of "prehistoric" micro-organisms *(Mollivirus Sibericum)).* The melting of permafrost (a natural geological phenomenon that refers to soils whose temperature remains below 0°C for at least two consecutive years) will facilitate human activity (soil exploitation, agriculture, etc.) and will be responsible for the release of pathogens such as Anthrax in the Yamal peninsula (Russia) in 2016, whereas the last recorded case was in 1941. Melting permafrost is also blamed for the Anthrax infection of 2,500 reindeer, 20 human cases including 1 death and 2,500 exposed in Siberia in 2016 (Ministry of Agriculture 2023) (Noël and publique France 2019, Miner, Turetsky et al. 2022, Ministry of Agriculture 2023).

Bird flu:

Several strains of highly pathogenic avian influenza virus are circulating around the world and in Europe. Outbreaks are regularly identified in poultry farms in Europe (e.g. H7N7 strain identified in April 2016 in a laying hen farm in Italy, numerous cases of highly pathogenic avian influenza in southwest France since late 2015, due to three strains: H5N1, H5N2 and H5N9). These viruses can be introduced into farms through trade. During periods of wild bird migration, the risk of infection of poultry farms is also increased (Sanguine 2021).

Fungal diseases:

Due to climate change, fungal pathogens or their vectors can spread geographically more widely, causing the emergence of diseases in regions where they had not previously been reported. floods, storms and hurricanes can disseminate and aerolize fungi or deposit them in traumatic wounds, leading to infections by previously unusual or unknown fungal species (Tazerji, Nardini et al. 2022).

Selection of antibiotic-resistant bacteria:

A study published in 2020 by scientists from IRD and CIRAD establishes for the first time the link between global warming and increased risk of antibiotic resistance in aquaculture. Their results show that global warming favors the development of pathogenic bacteria, and therefore the appearance of disease in aquaculture farms. This increased mortality prompts farmers to use more and more antibiotics, thus encouraging the emergence of resistant bacteria. The spread of resistant bacteria, or the transmission of their resistance genes to other non-resistant species capable of infecting humans or animals, is likely to lead to difficult diseases. In aquaculture, therefore, there is an urgent need to move towards production practices that are less dependent on antibiotics (Sanguine 2021).

2. Climate change and the emergence of wild reservoir diseases

Wildlife is considered one of the sources of emerging diseases. But within wildlife, emerging diseases are often detected as a result of increased mortality of a species and its adverse impact on biodiversity, or once the zoonotic potential of these diseases or their potential for transmission to domestic animals has been established (Barnouin and Sache 2010).

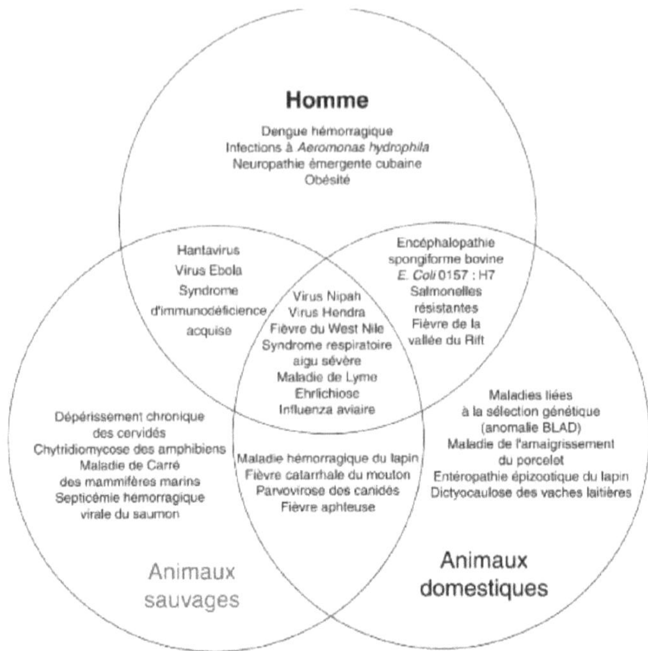

Figure 11: Examples of emerging diseases at the crossroads between domestic animals, wildlife and humans
(Barnouin and Sache 2010)

African swine fever

Western Europe (including Belgium) is free from classical swine fever. However, the virus is present in the wildlife of many Eastern European countries: wild boar represent a threat of introduction of the virus into the pig herd. From 2015 to 2019, several cases of the disease were discovered in domestic pigs in the European Union (Latvia, Lithuania, Estonia, Poland, Romania, Bulgaria and Sardinia). Since September 2018, African swine fever has been present in a wild boar population in the south of the Province of Luxembourg.

The wild boar population in these countries is also heavily affected. Measures are being taken at European level to limit the spread of the disease to western

Europe (Diricks 2018).

Rabies:

Rabies is endemic in many countries, with the exception of Australia and Antarctica, and is more prevalent in the developing countries of Africa and Asia due to a variety of factors, including rapid urbanization, a high volume of waste and a lack of adequate care (vaccination) and hygiene facilities. Rabies circulates through the urban cycle with interactions between domestic and stray dogs, and through the sylvatic cycle with interactions occurring between wild animals such as foxes, wolves, jackals, mongooses, raccoons, skunks and bats. These two cycles are interdependent and sometimes overlap. In developing and developed countries, dogs and wildlife respectively are the main causes of rabies transmission. It has been shown that various social and environmental factors play an important role in the contact between domestic animals and wildlife, with urbanization, deforestation and waste accumulation being the most important of these, leading to the emergence and re-emergence of rabies in rabies-free areas (Tazerji, Nardini et al. 2022).

Ebola disease:

The Ebola virus belongs to the *FHoviridae* family. The Ebolavirus genus *contains* five distinct species: Zaire Ebolavirus (EBOV), Suda Ebolavirus (SUDV), Tai Forest Ebolavirus, Bundibugyo Ebolavirus (BDBV) and Reston Ebolavirus. EBOV, SUDV and BDBV have caused epidemics of Ebola virus disease in Central and West Africa, with increased frequency and case-fatality rates ranging from 30% to 90% in humans. Bombali virus (BOMV), a new Ebola virus belonging to the proposed new species, has recently been detected in bats in Sierra Leon and Kenya. Mengla virus (MLAV) has also been discovered in fruit bats in China. Olivero et al (Olivero, Fa et al. 2020), studied the effect of anthropogenic actions on Ebola emergence and proposed that there is a significant link between forest degradation and fragmentation and human Ebola epidemics. Deforestation has the potential to alter the abundance, composition and perhaps exposure behavior of reservoir species. As a result, interaction between infected animals and humans is increased (Tazerji, Nardini et al. 2022).

Leptospirosis:

The intrusion of wild species into cities increases the potential risk of *Leptospira* transmission. Wild boar, foxes, deer, skunks and raccoons can be frequently seen not only in suburbs, but also sometimes in older urban neighborhoods in some countries. In a study carried out in Berlin, *Leptospira* was isolated from 18% of suburban wild boars (Jansen, Luge et al. 2007, Tazerji, Nardini et al. 2022).

It's also important to note that legal and illegal international trade in exotic animals is growing strongly (in 2006: 4 million birds, 650,000 reptiles, 40,000 primates...), with an increased risk of spreading exotic pathogens (Angot 2009).

3. Climate change and disease emergence due to vector redistribution

Climate change can also modify pathogen cycles, leading to more rapid growth outside the host and prolonged seasonal presence. Ticks, for example, hematophagous ectoparasites, are normally active in spring and autumn, and inactive in winter. Milder winters would lead to their longer persistence in the outdoor environment (even continuous in some countries of the world), with a greater risk of contamination by the diseases they carry (piroplasmosis, Lyme disease) (French Ministry of Agriculture 2023) (Miner, Turetsky et al. 2022, French Ministry of Agriculture 2023).

3.1. Tick-borne diseases

Climate and other environmental changes are expected to increase the risk associated with ticks and tick-borne diseases. The prevalence, activity and geographical range of a number of ticks and the pathogens they carry are also expected to increase. This is due to meteorological changes which are also causing an increase in the geographical range of breeding and reservoir animals. Rising temperatures have improved conditions for tick survival and reproduction, and increased the speed of their development. As a result, their life cycle has accelerated. The consequences of this phenomenon are an increase in tick abundance where they were already present, the spread of tick populations to higher latitudes, and an increase in tick activity and foraging, leading to prolonged seasonal activity. Animals that are reservoir hosts and breeding hosts play a crucial role in the transmission cycle of tick-borne pathogens and the life cycle of ticks, respectively. The reservoir host is the source of the pathogen for the immature stages of ticks. The main reservoir host in most tick-borne diseases are wild rodents, including mice. Breeding hosts are the source of blood meals essential for reproduction in adult females. Climate change affects both the breeding and reservoir hosts involved in the tick life cycle and the transmission of tick-borne diseases, respectively. Rising temperatures will lead to an expansion of the territory occupied by rodents, as well as an increase in their abundance and activity (Bouchard, Dibernardo et al. 2019).

Several diseases are expected to emerge as a result of these changes: Crimean Congo fever, Lyme disease, babesiosis, anaplasmosis (Bouchard, Dibernardo et al. 2019).

Crimean-Congo hemorrhagic fever:

The Crimean Congo hemorrhagic fever virus belongs to the *Orthonairovirus* genus *and the Nairoviridae family.* The disease is endemic in Africa, the Balkans, the Middle East and Asia. After infection, animals show no clinical signs, but it causes severe hemorrhagic fever in humans, with a case-fatality rate of up to 40%. The absence of symptoms in animals makes this disease difficult to detect.

Over the past few years, researchers have noted the progressive establishment in southern France of the tick *(Hyalomma marginatum)* responsible for transmitting this virus. In 2018, antibodies were found in cattle and small ruminants in Corsica, without the virus being formally identified. The Crimean Congo hemorrhagic fever virus has never yet been detected in France, although a strain of the virus was identified in Spain causing the first human cases in the region in 2016,2018 and 2020 (Sanguine 2021).

In Tunisia, three studies have examined the presence of antibodies to Crimean Congo hemorrhagic fever virus (CCHF) in domestic animal sera in recent years (Rekik, Hammami et al. 2024).

The study by Khamassi Khbou et al, carried out on 270 sera from Tunisian sheep from different regions of the country and analyzed by ELISA, showed a seroprevalence of 1.1% (Khamassi Khbou, Romdhane et al. 2021).

Zouaghi et al. (2021) reported in a study carried out in northern Tunisia (governorates of Ariana, Beja, Bizerte, Jendouba, Kef, Nabeul, Tunis and Zaghouan), using ELISA and indirect immunofluorescence assay (IIFAT), an overall seroprevalence of 6.2% (20/235) in sheep, 7.8% (13/166) in goats and 11.1% (43/388) in cattle (Zouaghi, Bouattour et al. 2021)

A cross-sectional survey was conducted by Bouaicha et al. on 273 dromedary sera from the governorate of Tataouine, southern Tunisia, using both the ID Screen-French ELISA multispecies FHCC double antigen test and ELISA in Tunisian dromedaries *(Camelus dromedarius)* yielded a surprisingly high seroprevalence; of 89.7% (245/273) (Bouaicha, Eisenbarth et al. 2021)

3.2. Mosquito-borne diseases

The report of the United Nations Intergovernmental Panel on Climate Change indicates that mosquito-borne diseases are the infectious diseases most sensitive to climate change. The main aspects of climate change affecting endemic mosquitoes are temperature rises and fluctuations in precipitation (Ludwig, Zheng et al. 2019).

Rising average temperatures are not the only factor affecting the range of vector-borne diseases: for mosquito-borne diseases in particular, rainfall is a determining factor. More abundant rainfall generally increases the potential extent of mosquito breeding sites and breeding grounds in the environment. The relationship is often non-linear. Above-average rainfall generally makes mosquitoes more abundant by giving them access to more standing water, while excessive or violent rainfall can wash away and destroy eggs, and drive out larvae living in selected habitats. Thus, species of the *Aedes* and *Culex* genera thrive on high accumulations of precipitation (corresponding to the start of rainy seasons), followed by several hydration/dehydration cycles. (Ludwig, Zheng et al. 2019, Dungu and Anyamba 2020, Ministry of Agriculture 2023).

High temperatures can accelerate mosquito development at immature stages of the life cycle, leading to higher reproduction rates and exponential population growth. These high temperatures reduce the extrinsic incubation period, so that infected mosquitoes become infectious sooner; for example, outbreaks of West Nile virus infection appear to occur more frequently in Canada when seasonal temperatures are above average, as these conditions favor rapid virus acquisition in mosquito vectors and prolong host-seeking by potentially infected female mosquitoes. It has been reported that in Korea and Japan, the length of the transmission season can be extended by several months when average summer temperatures rise by as little as 5°C. Changes in rainfall increase the availability of stagnant water, where mosquitoes lay their eggs and where immature mosquitoes live. Consequently, these changes have a strong impact on mosquito reproduction (Chevalier, Courtin et al. 2015, Ludwig, Zheng et al. 2019).

Climate change is also expected to affect disease transmission through several mechanisms:

- Reduced egg development time in newly-fed adult female mosquitoes, resulting in shorter blood-meal intervals and more frequent feedings
- Reduction in the length of the extrinsic incubation period, and therefore the time required for mosquitoes to become carriers of infection
- Increased lifespan of mosquitoes leading to more bites by individuals carrying infections (Ng, Rees et al. 2019)

It is well known that mosquito-borne diseases are sensitive to climate, and that climatic conditions determine the geographical limits and seasonality of transmission. Climate change therefore has an effect on the emergence and establishment of exotic (previously non-existent in a country) mosquito-borne diseases. When the vector is present, climate change is likely to increase the number of cases of exotic mosquito-borne diseases contracted abroad by amplifying the natural transmission cycle and the probability of vector/reservoir/human-animal contact in the country of origin. They are also likely to enable sustainable indigenous transmission in the short term (Githeko, Lindsay et al. 2001, Cheung, Sarmiento et al. 2013, Ng, Rees et al. 2019).

The various species of mosquito have different characteristics in terms of their preferred habitats and pathogenic load. Due to climate change, the prevalence of West Nile virus and Eastern Equine Encephalitis (EEE) and California serogroup viruses, could gain in importance (Ludwig, Zheng et al. 2019).

West Nile fever:

West Nile fever is caused by a *Flavivirus* that has long been known on many continents, and wild birds are its essential reservoirs. Infected birds develop sufficient viremia to allow infection of vectors (mainly mosquitoes of the *Cuiex* genus). In Europe, the disease has been observed in human cases in Romania (1996 to 1997) and the Czech Republic (1997). Equine cases were reported in Italy (1998) and France (2000). The emergence of West Nile fever in European countries should not be ruled out, given the historical example of its appearance ten years ago in NewYork (Brugère-Picoux and Chomel 2009).

Bluetongue (Blue tongue disease) (*Bluetongue* :

FCO is caused by an *orbivirus* transmitted by a biting arthropod of the *Culicoides* genus*: Cuiicoides imicoia.* This ruminant-specific disease was considered exotic in Europe until 1998, despite a few outbreaks in the Iberian Peninsula. Since then, of the twenty-four known serotypes of the FCO virus, eight (serotypes 1, 2, 4, 6, 8, 9, 11, 16) have circulated in Europe. The biggest surprise was the emergence of serotype 8 in 2006 in several regions: Belgium, Germany, the Netherlands, France and Luxembourg for having been considered a risk zone. What's more, prior to this epizootic, FCO was known as a serious disease in sheep, whereas serotype 8, whose origin is still unknown, also proved pathogenic in cattle and goats. Then, in 2008, another serotype (serotype 1) spread from Spain, forcing the implementation of a mass herd vaccination campaign in 2009 to combat this infection, which had long been a notifiable disease. The arrival of FCO in Europe illustrates that the distribution area of disease vectors is never definitive. This fever, an arbovirosis of ruminants widely distributed in the intertropical zone, was considered an exotic disease in Europe until the late 1990s. Over the past two decades, it has spread not only to countries around the Mediterranean, but also to Northern Europe, creating a major health and economic crisis. To immunize its cattle and sheep populations, Belgium launched a vaccination campaign in April 2016. In 2014 and 2015, several European Union member states (Greece, Italy, Hungary, Romania, Bulgaria, Cyprus, Croatia, Serbia, Bosnia-Herzegovina) and other border territories (Turkey, the Balkans) were affected by a serotype 4 virus. Since March 2019, serotype 8 has again been present in Belgium (Brugère-Picoux and Chomel 2009, Chevalier, Courtin et al. 2015).

Rift Valley fever:

Rift Valley fever (RVF), so named because it was first described in Kenya in 1931, is a mosquito-borne zoonosis affecting livestock (especially sheep) and humans. It is caused by a *Phlebovirus* of the *Bunyaviridae* family, found in blood and nasal secretions. Rainy periods favor the proliferation of vectors (Aedesen in particular, *Culex...}* and the main factors in the spread of RVF are the movements of infected domestic animals. The virus has been isolated from numerous wild animal species, in particular African buffalo, which may play a role in the natural infection cycle. The disease is one of the most serious, periodically and severely affecting both humans and livestock in sub-Saharan Africa. Transmission of the disease to humans occurs during enzootic or epizootic outbreaks in sheep, cattle, goats and camels, either via vectors or through contact with the animals, notably during parturition, slaughter of infected animals and autopsy of deceased animals, or even through ingestion of contaminated raw milk. The map below (fig. 12) shows that the regional epicentres of RVF outbreaks are located in eastern and southern Africa. These epicenters are modulated by rainfall variability associated with the El Niño and La Niña phases of the El Niño phenomenon. Known in sub-Saharan Africa, RVF has demonstrated its ability to cross geographical barriers such as the Sahara, the Red Sea and the Indian Ocean, following the appearance of outbreaks in recent decades in Egypt, the Arabian Peninsula, Madagascar and Mayotte, in most cases as a result of animal movements (mainly small ruminants). The first outbreak outside Africa in 2000, in Saudi Arabia and then Yemen, followed the importation of infected animals from Kenya and Somalia after unusually high rainfall had boosted the mosquito population. Following this episode, in 2006 and 2007, severe epidemics occurred in East Africa after heavy rainfall. Depending on the geographical area affected, RVF epidemic waves depend on the complex interaction between rainfall, vector reproduction possibilities (with or without transovarial transmission of the virus) and host receptivity. RVF is a matter of concern for all those involved in animal and human health, as the presence of potential vectors means that there is a risk of it spreading to other, hitherto unscathed, geographical areas such as Europe, Asia and the Americas. The Maghreb countries are in the front line, in particular due to the large number of little or uncontrolled exchanges of small ruminants via trans-Saharan routes with neighboring countries. The density of passenger traffic between southern European countries (as well as the clandestine import of sheep) could allow RVF to be transferred from a Maghreb country to Europe, particularly France. There is growing interest in this pathogen as a potential bioterrorism agent (Brugère-Picoux and Chomel 2009, Ludwig, Zheng et al. 2019, Dungu and Anyamba 2020).

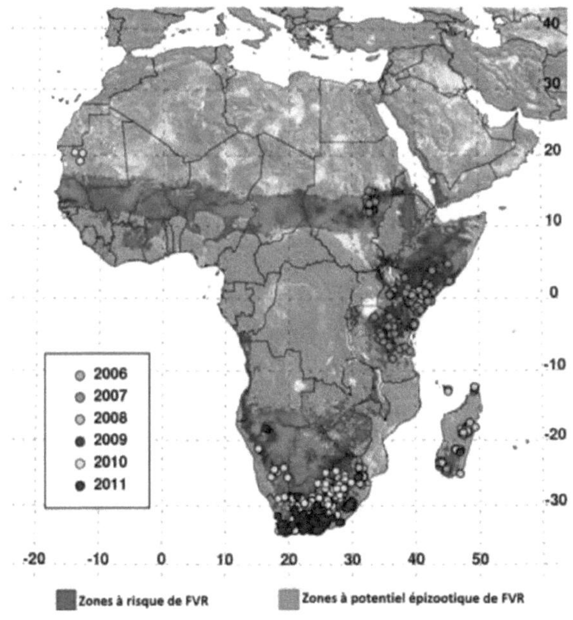

Figure 12: Composite map showing the risk of Rift Valley fever, with areas at risk in red and the location of various outbreaks between 2006 and 2011.

. (Dungu and Anyamba 2020)

Tunisia is considered to be at high risk of RVF spread due to its location, climatic and environmental characteristics, the abundance of vectors transmitting the RVF virus, and the presence of animal species at risk for this disease. Various serological surveys were carried out on livestock, some of which proved negative, while others showed seropositivity levels of 0.17% and 34% respectively. In public health, a serological study in central-eastern Tunisia showed seropositivity in patients with unexplained febrile syndrome and in slaughterhouse workers. A serological survey conducted by the Tunisian health watch center in December 2018-December 2019 on 1,025 dromedaries in southern Tunisia revealed a single seropositive dromedary (0.07%). Selmi et al. in 2020 found 162 positive responses among 470 ELISA-tested dromedary sera. These two studies show that Tunisian dromedaries have been exposed to this virus and could contribute to its dissemination among farmers and other livestock.
(Hassine, Amdouni et al. 2017, Selmi, Mamlouk et al. 2020, Ben Ali and al 2022)

Lumpy skin disease:

This disease is caused by a virus and affects mainly dairy cattle. It is characterized by large nodules on the skin and mucous membranes. It is transmitted mainly by insects. Outbreaks were observed in 2016 in Turkey, Greece, Bulgaria and Macedonia. These countries have organized vaccination campaigns to bring the disease under control. The disease is currently spreading (fig.13) in the Middle East, the Near East, south-eastern Europe and the northern Caucasus, as well as in North Africa (fig.14).

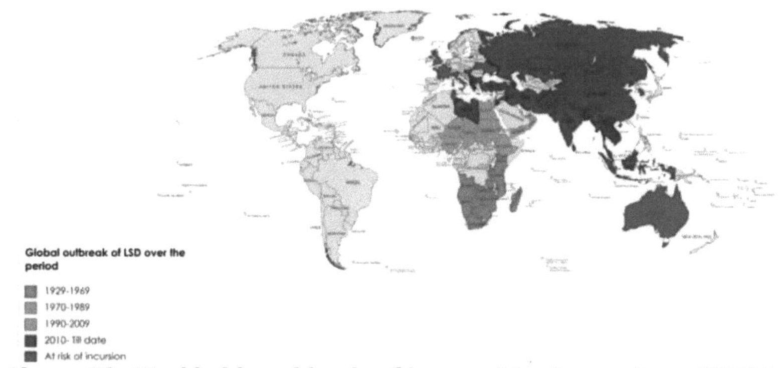

Figure 13: Worldwide epidemic of lumpy skin disease from 1929 to 2023

(Akther, Akter et al. 2023).

A rapid and uncontrollable spread of the disease has highlighted, in many cases, the lack of preparedness of the livestock sector and Veterinary Authorities in the face of the disease (Tuppurainen and Galon 2016, Das, Chowdhury et al. 2021). Lumpy skin disease was first reported in Tunisia on August 14, 2024, in the northwestern region of Firnana (fig.25).

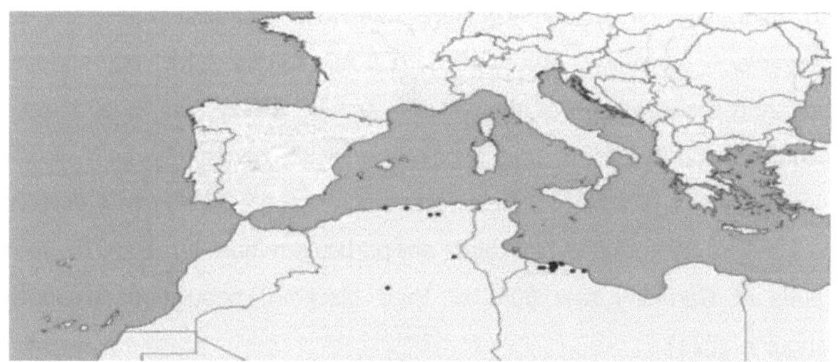

Figure 14: Distribution of outbreaks of lumpy skin disease in North Africa

January to August 2024 (Perrin, Limon-Vega et al. 2024)

Leishmaniasis:

Climate change can have an impact by altering environments and ecosystems, and with it the habitats of many animals and their parasites and pathogens. The effects of climate change can modify the distribution of leishmaniasis in three ways: directly through the effect of temperature on the parasite and on the development and competence of vectors, and indirectly through the effect of temperature and other environmental variables on the distribution and abundance of sandflies, which affect the amount of human and animal contact with the transmission cycle (Tazerji, Nardini et al. 2022).

The Utusu virus:

The Usutu virus was first detected in France in 2015. From June to September, scientists spotted it at several sites in mosquitoes of *the Culexpipiens* species, common in France, and with high prevalences (more than one in ten mosquitoes). In 2016, two strains of the virus moved to Europe. One caused a human case in Montpellier, and the other caused severe bird mortality. Usutu has an ecology similar to that of West Nile fever. It arrives in Europe with migratory birds, and circulates between animals thanks to the *Culexpipiens* mosquito. Since 2015, CIRAD teams have been closely monitoring the evolution of this virus in France. Every year, they capture mosquitoes and look for the presence of the virus. The Usutu virus is capable of infecting over fifty bird species, spread across more than twenty different bird families. Raptors and blackbirds are particularly hard hit. In 2018, some regions of Germany saw 60% of their blackbird populations disappear (Sanguine 2021).

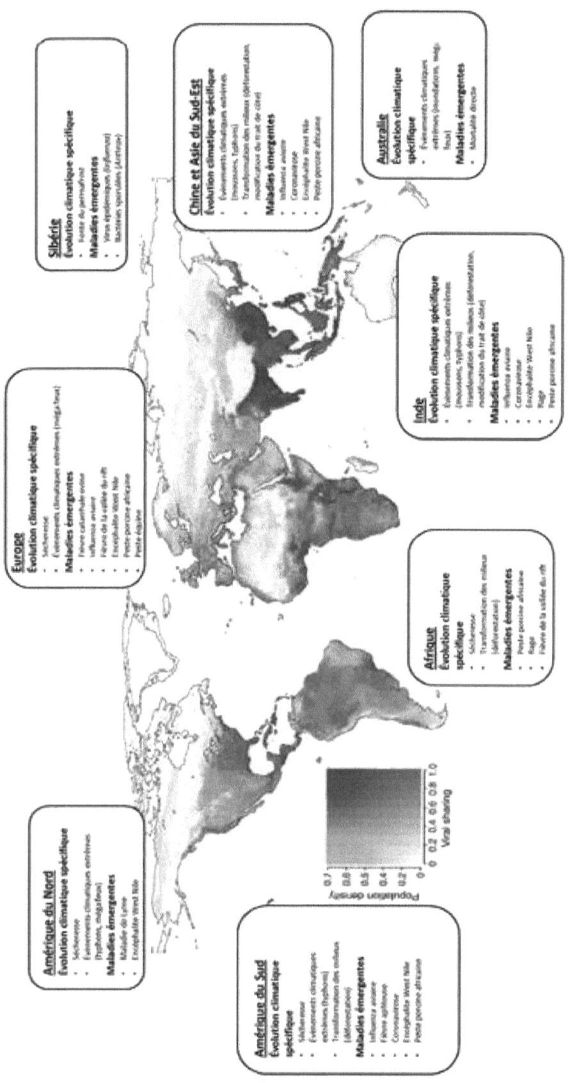

Figure 15: Major emerging diseases in different regions of the world for which a correlation with climate change has been established

(Carlson, Albery et al. 2022, Ministry of Agriculture 2023).

The coloring corresponds to an index of the risk of emergence of viral diseases transmissible between species, taking into account population densities and the inter-transmissibility of locally circulating viruses. The regions most at risk are shown in violet/indigo.

B. Impact of emerging diseases

Such emerging diseases can have a major impact on animal health, for example if they spread very rapidly from one herd to another, causing an epidemic, or if they cause significant mortality and/or economic losses. They can also have an impact on public health if they are zoonoses, i.e. animal diseases transmissible to humans. Examples of zoonotic animal diseases include avian flu, brucellosis, tuberculosis and rabies. Emerging diseases have economic repercussions that go far beyond their immediate health costs. Their appearance can lead to a slowdown in trade and travel, or cause a disproportionate sense of alarm, particularly if rumors spread of intentional use. To contain the threat posed by these diseases on an international scale, we need to ensure that surveillance and response are well coordinated at global level. In the event of contagious animal disease epidemics, control and eradication measures, such as vaccination campaigns, are costly at the collective level. The economic consequences can run into the hundreds of millions of euros. Concrete examples are mad cow disease, blue tongue disease, foot-and-mouth disease, bird flu, etc. An estimated 17% of livestock production yield is lost due to animal diseases in developed countries, and much more in developing countries (Diricks 2018, WHO 2024).

I. Animal level :

Climate change can have a direct impact on animal physiology: droughts and heat waves cause heat stress, leading to suffering, dehydration and cardio-respiratory disorders, which can be fatal. These effects manifest themselves in weight loss, reproductive disorders and behavioral changes, which in the long term threaten the general health of animal populations and can alter the productive yields of livestock. The main repercussions of climate change felt at animal level are changes in natural habitat and diet (quantity and type of feed) (fig.16). Environmental constraints and poor nutrition severely limit animal productivity, especially in developing countries. Weakened animals are all the more prone to disease. Non-transmissible diseases (metabolic or reproductive disorders) can thus be a direct consequence of weather conditions, themselves impacted by climate change. In the case of livestock, these effects can be reinforced by the quantitative and qualitative alteration of animal feed during extreme weather events (drought, heatwaves, floods).

Climate change is also having an impact on the food intake of wild animals, which are finding it difficult to feed due to changes in plant cover or the disappearance of certain prey. As a result, they have to move outside their usual territory (fig.17), even into areas occupied by domestic animals or humans. The resulting contacts can be the source of contamination.

The consequences of endemic diseases are felt by animals in terms of animal welfare and biodiversity, with the result that some species are decimated by endemic diseases to the point of becoming endangered species. (Leboucq 2019, Wright 2022, Ministry of Agriculture 2023).

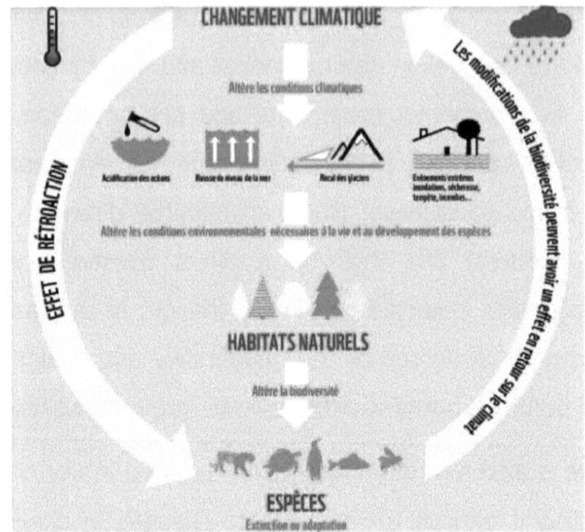

Figure 16: Impact of climate change on animals

(Valingot, Chaumien et al. 2015)

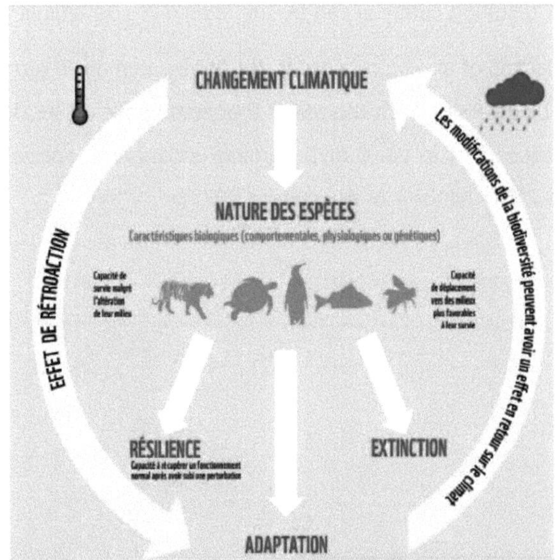

Figure 17: Impact of climate change on animals

(Valingot, Chaumien et al. 2015)

II. At the operating level

At farm level, good animal health ensures animal welfare and good animal production (livestock, meat, milk, etc.), and is an element of economic prosperity for livestock farmers. Livestock accounts for 40% of the value of agriculture worldwide. They provide income and livelihoods for one in five people, mainly in developing countries (Huntington, Bernardo et al. 2021).

However, animal diseases can considerably reduce this potential. Depending on the severity and type of disease, they can have negative consequences.

The installation of an infectious disease on a farm leads to additional costs, a drop in production, fertility problems and abortions, mortality, and so on. This leads to direct economic loss, which in turn can have major social consequences.

Contagious animal diseases can also result in farm sequestration, i.e. a ban on transporting and marketing animals, or even slaughter. They also have consequences for national and international trade and exports. All this has direct and indirect economic consequences for livestock farmers (Tab.2).

Table II: Direct and indirect consequences of emerging diseases at farm level

(Huntington, Bernardo et al. 2021)

Direct economic impact	Indirect economic impact
Animal mortality	Reduced fertility
Low yields (lower milk production)	Changes in animal population structure
Treatment costs (antibiotics, insecticides, etc.)	Rising labor costs
Vaccines	Deferral of sales of animals and animal by-products Limited access to markets

In all cases, the direct costs of animal diseases are directly linked to the speed with which outbreaks are contained: case studies show that the speed with which an outbreak is diagnosed and appropriate measures implemented is decisive in keeping direct losses to a minimum. Conversely, inappropriate control and eradication measures are at the root of endemic situations, which are much more difficult and infinitely more costly to control and eradicate.

Consumers quickly lose confidence when it comes to diseases that can be transmitted to humans via food. This can cause the market to collapse, with economic consequences for breeders (Diricks 2018).

III. At national level :

Climate change is altering the nature and likelihood of animal disease outbreaks in a given region. For example, epizootics caused by vector-borne diseases have become more frequent, and now affect a wider geographical area. However, health risks still vary from one region to another. In addition to this disparity, the actual consequences vary according to the characteristics of the food system under consideration.

The greatest impact is seen in low- and middle-income countries, which are generally more vulnerable due to their lower capacity to monitor animal diseases and implement animal health operations to deal with them. However, more than just the level of national income, it is above all the characteristics of the local food system (particularly in terms of animal population density) that condition the consequences of global warming (intensity and nature of effects). In regions with intensive, large-scale livestock farming, an epizootic can take on a wide scope and have considerable macroeconomic impacts: epizootic outbreaks are favored by the concentration of individuals, and management includes restrictive measures (movement bans, sometimes accompanied by downgrading of health status as defined by the World Organization for Animal Health (OIE), culling). The entire agricultural and commercial sector may be affected. In regions where subsistence family farming predominates, diseases often persist in an endemic form that can lead to crises. Only infected farms are then impacted (illness or death of animals leading to economic losses) (Thornton, Jones et al. 2010, Leboucq 2019, Ministère de l'agriculture 2023).

IV. Internationally :

The health crises of bovine spongiform encephalopathy, West Nile fever and Highly Pathogenic Avian Influenza (HPAI) show that emerging diseases can take on global importance in the space of a few years, months or even weeks. The intensity and speed of intra- and inter-continental transport, as well as more subtle factors such as the panzootic spread of HPAI and the homogeneity of the avian strains used on poultry farms worldwide, explain this rapidity and underline the need for a global response to the threat, in terms of both management and research. These factors represent multiple challenges for societies in both the South and the North.

The economic impact of emerging diseases is high, with direct costs (clinical impact, economic impact, public health impact, cost of surveillance and control) and/or indirect costs (disruption of dietary balances, restriction or prohibition of national and international trade, lack of sales due to consumer distrust) (Camus and Lancelot 2007).

The main examples illustrating the impact at international level are :

* African swine fever: The declaration of numerous outbreaks in Europe cost between 1 and 2 billion euros, with economic repercussions in the region. It has led to a 10% drop in world pork supply, due to the concentration of the sector in Asia. The persistence of the infectious agent in wild boar makes control of the disease difficult (Huntington, Bernardo et al. 2021).

*H1N1 influenza: Panic and misinformation led to unnecessary pig slaughter and economic losses.

*Influenza H5N1: This is the cause of a global economic and food shock, given that the poultry sector is the major supplier of animal and human food, catering and tourism (Huntington, Bernardo et al. 2021).

* Bovine spongiform encephalopathy: This has led to changes in animal feed regulations and caused major economic losses in the beef sector in the UK and worldwide (Huntington, Bernardo et al. 2021).

Part 3: Prevention of emerging diseases

I. The role of international bodies

A proactive approach is essential, and for this the world needs well-trained, operational professionals - biologists, ecologists, microbiologists, modelers, doctors and veterinarians.

The World Organization for Animal Health (OIE) is the international reference body for animal health. Since its creation, WHOA has played a key role as the only international reference organization dedicated to animal health, benefiting from proven international recognition and direct collaboration with the Veterinary Services of all Member Countries. Because of the close relationship between animal health and animal protection, WHOA has become, at the request of its Member Countries, the leading international organization in the field of animal protection. WOSHA works closely with FAO and WHO, as well as with the World Bank and regional organizations such as the European Commission (WOSHA 2024).

All these bodies are working towards the same general objective, which is to reduce the impact of climate change on animal health and the spread of infectious diseases. Fields of action :

- Strengthen and extend the platforms, infrastructures and tools developed at global and national level to prevent, prepare for and respond to animal health emergencies triggered by climate change.

- Develop epidemiological surveillance capabilities for diseases and their vectors.

- Promote research to model and predict the impact of climate change on the spread of infectious diseases (FAO 2020).

1. Role of the World Organization for Animal Health (OIE)

The surveillance and control of animal epidemics (epizootics) is based on actions to be taken at local, national, regional and global levels, based on guidelines defined at world level. The development of these standards is one of the mandates assigned to the World Organization for Animal Health (OIE) (Angot 2009).

WHO is the world's authority on animal health. Founded in 1924 as the Office International des Épizooties (OIE), it adopted the common name of World Organization for Animal Health in May 2003. It currently has 183 member countries. As an intergovernmental organization, it is committed to the transparent dissemination of information on animal diseases, and to improving animal health worldwide, thereby building a safer, healthier and more sustainable world. (WHOA 2024).

The main objective of WHOA's mission is "To improve animal health on a global scale, thus ensuring a better future for all". To achieve this, WHOA carries out the following missions:

- Transparency: guaranteeing transparency of the animal disease situation worldwide; each member country undertakes to declare any animal diseases it detects on its territory. WHOA then disseminates the information to all other countries, so that they can protect themselves. This information also concerns diseases transmissible to humans. It is disseminated as a matter of urgency or on a delayed basis, depending on the severity of the disease. These surveillance and monitoring objectives apply to both natural and intentional health events. Dissemination media include e-mail, Health Information and the WAHIS global health information database interface.

- Scientific information: Collecting, analyzing and disseminating veterinary scientific information; WHOA collects and analyzes all new scientific information relating to animal disease control. It then provides this information to Member Countries to help them improve the methods they use to control and eradicate these diseases. Guidelines are prepared for this purpose by WHOA's network of 246 Collaborating Centres and Reference

Laboratories around the world.

Scientific information is also disseminated through various books and periodicals published by OMSA, notably the Revue scientifique et technique (3 issues per year).

- International solidarity: providing expertise and stimulating international solidarity to control animal diseases; WHOA provides technical support to Member Countries wishing to support operations to control and eradicate animal diseases, including those transmissible to humans. In particular, WHOA offers its expertise to the poorest countries to help them control animal diseases that cause losses to their livestock, can endanger public health and threaten other Member Countries. At regional and national level, WHOA maintains constant contact with international financial organizations, to persuade them to invest more and better in the control of animal diseases and zoonoses.

- Sanitary safety: To guarantee the safety of world trade by drawing up sanitary standards for international trade in animals and animal products, within the framework of the mandate given to WHOA by the World Trade Organization (WTO) SPS Agreement; WHOA draws up normative documents concerning the rules that can be used by member countries to protect themselves from the introduction of diseases and pathogens, without creating unjustified sanitary barriers. The main standard-setting documents produced by WHOA are : The Terrestrial Animal Health Code, the Manual of Standards for Diagnostic Tests and Vaccines, the International Aquatic Animal Health Code and the Diagnostic Manual for Aquatic Animal Diseases.

WHOA standards are recognized by the World Trade Organization as international health standards. They are drawn up by elected Specialized Commissions and Working Groups comprising the world's leading scientists, most of whom are experts from the network of some 246 Collaborating

Centres and Reference Laboratories, which also contribute to the scientific objectives of WHOA. These standards are adopted by the World Assembly of Delegates.

- Promoting Veterinary Services: Promoting the legal framework and resources of Veterinary Services; Veterinary Services and laboratories in developing countries and countries in transition urgently need support in order to be equipped with the infrastructure, resources and capacities to enable their countries to better reap the benefits of the WTO Agreement on the Application of Sanitary and Phytosanitary Measures (SPS Agreement) and to better protect animal and public health.

WHOA considers Veterinary Services to be an International Public Good, and bringing them up to international standards (structure, organization, resources, capacities, role of paraprofessionals) to be a priority for public investment.

- Food safety and animal welfare: Better guarantee food safety and promote animal welfare using a scientific approach; WHOA member countries have decided to better guarantee the safety of food of animal origin by strengthening synergies between the activities of WHOA and those of the Codex Alimentarius Commission. WOSHA's standard-setting activities in this field are focused on the prevention of hazards existing before animals are slaughtered or their products (meat, milk, eggs, etc.) are first processed, which may subsequently generate risks for consumers (WOSHA 2024).

2. Role of the United Nations (FAO)

As part of a collaboration between the Food and Agriculture Organization of the United Nations (FAO) and the United States Agency for International Development (USAID), the FAO provided technical training covering a wide range of skills, including disease forecasting and surveillance, laboratory work, biosecurity, prevention and control methods, and strategies for dealing with epidemics. In all, 3,266 veterinarians in Asia, 619 in West Africa, 459 in East Africa and 363 in the Middle East benefited from these training courses to combat the emergence of new diseases, by tackling the source directly (United Nations 2018).

II. Controlling and managing emerging diseases

Controlling the spread of an infectious disease in a population requires precise knowledge of how the agent in question is transmitted, whether natural reservoirs exist, and the characteristics of the vectors involved (Shongo, Lubala et al. 2020).

Indeed, these diseases often originate in the South and threaten or arrive in the North, without borders. Avian influenza is a good illustration of the global dimension of certain diseases, and the need for a global approach. The most effective control measures are those that target the sources. On the one hand, protecting ourselves in the countries of the North means supporting the countries of the South, so that they can control these diseases. Research, particularly epidemiological research, also requires North/South partnerships. On the other hand, it is important to develop new diagnostic tests and vaccines that are not only effective but also more "robust", less costly and more reliable for use in the difficult conditions encountered in developing countries (Camus and Lancelot 2007).

For better management of emergencies, we need information systems that can act in real time, and whose features are dedicated to the detection and epidemiological analysis of clinical emergence (Barnouin and Sache 2010).

1. Screening and early diagnosis

As far as early clinical diagnosis is concerned, the aim is to rapidly detect and document two main types of situation that could represent an outbreak. The first type concerns the appearance of "atypical syndromes", i.e. syndromes whose clinical picture is not attributable to a listed disease, or is attributable to a known disease, but presenting at least one of the following characteristics: pathology not known in the region of emergence, not known in the species affected, of exceptional or recurrent severity (virus creating immunodeficiency and favoring the development of recurrent bacterial infections). In practice, the detection of an atypical syndrome may correspond either to a new pathology, or to a rare or poorly documented disease "brought to light" by greater attention to atypia (in particular, following the introduction of specific vigilance). The second type of clinical situation to be taken into account for early detection of emergences concerns listed diseases that we choose to monitor a priori because we suspect their emergence via an increase (apparent or foreseeable) in their incidence; this is either based on preliminary observations, or because the environmental factors or husbandry practices linked to the disease have recently undergone, or are likely to undergo, changes that could lead to an increase in the disease's incidence (tick-borne diseases : Lyme disease, ehrlichiosis; diseases vectorized by mosquitoes or Culicoides: West Nile, Blue Tongue) (Barnouin and VOURC'H 2004).

The breeder is the first link in the detection chain, and is usually the one to notice the first changes and clinical signs. Here are a few examples of unusual signs or behaviors that will attract the breeder's attention and that he or she should communicate to the veterinarian:

- Any signs of disease or unusual behavior observed in your animals, i.e. that you have never seen before (e.g. bleeding, trembling, paralysis, etc.), or any mortality that exceeds the usual threshold;

- Abortions or fertility problems;

- An abnormal drop in food intake, daily weight gain or milk production.

Practicing veterinarians, along with livestock farmers, are the key players in monitoring the outbreak of emerging animal diseases. Because they are in daily contact with animals on the farm, they are the first to notice unusual clinical signs and to take the necessary measures in time, before the disease spreads and an epidemic breaks out. They also have a key role to play in transmitting information between breeders and the competent authorities, and in centralizing information. This centralization makes it possible to identify the evolution of new diseases at an early stage, enabling them to be managed appropriately (Barnouin and VOURC'H 2004, Diricks 2019).

2. Traceability

Animal identification and traceability are extremely useful tools for the effective control of animal diseases. When new outbreaks occur, these measures facilitate the identification of animals and animal products potentially exposed to the pathogen, and enable them to be traced, so that appropriate control measures can be implemented.

In the event of the introduction of an emerging animal disease, a key factor in limiting its spread is the rapid identification of its source, i.e. the animal or herd that caused it (upstream traceability). Indeed, it is in this way that it will be possible to identify, thanks to the various documents and certificates, to which herds these animals may have spread the disease (downstream traceability). This is particularly important at the start of an epidemic, when the number of affected herds is still low and there is still a chance of containing the epidemic. This traceability requires rigorous maintenance of documents relating to animal movements and animal identification (OIE 2015, Diricks 2018).

2. Epidemiological surveillance

Effective surveillance, whether active (planned) or passive (based on event detection), is a prerequisite for any action to prevent and control animal diseases. WHO defines surveillance as "the systematic and continuous collection, compilation and analysis of data, and their dissemination in a time frame compatible with the implementation of the necessary measures" (OIE

Terrestrial Animal Health Code). To be effective, this strategy presupposes optimal communication and collaboration between all stakeholders, at all levels of the animal production chain; that is, from the farmer, his veterinarian and the local laboratory, to the highest national veterinary authorities (OIE 2015).

Epidemiological cycles, determinants and circumstances of emergence, and control methods are insufficiently understood and mastered. Ecological and epidemiological approaches using a range of modeling tools can help us to understand complex epidemiologies, and to use predictive models to assist decision-making in terms of surveillance and control. Knowledge of the epidemiological system is necessary, but not sufficient: we need to design and implement surveillance methods capable of detecting the appearance of new diseases or an abnormal increase in the frequency of known diseases. It is then necessary to assess the capacity of local, regional and national authorities, as well as health systems, to become involved in surveillance, and then to implement control measures in a rapid, coherent and concerted manner (Camus and Lancelot 2007).

Improved epidemiological surveillance of infectious diseases is essential in this fight. Collaboration with the veterinary community is essential: several "One Health" programs have been set up to help developing countries, strengthening their overall response capacity. Technology can also play a major role in predicting emergence. For example, the use of satellite imagery can detect changes in vegetation patterns in response to rainfall. The use of satellite photos taken over East Africa, for example, makes it possible to predict Rift Valley fever epidemics in cattle, a consequence of increased vector activity. Crucial aspects in the control of any new epidemic include its early recognition, good access to diagnostic facilities, and the dissemination and analysis of surveillance data (Choumet 2021).

For vector-borne diseases (arboviruses), it is more appropriate to monitor risks in vector populations than to wait for cases to appear in animals and humans. The World Health Organization has stressed the importance of identifying and monitoring various vector populations as part of global surveillance, including mosquitoes that can carry and transmit arboviruses (Ludwig, Zheng et al. 2019).

3. Importance of continuing education

In order to remain attentive and vigilant, to easily recognize unusual signs of emerging animal diseases and to detect them early, it is essential to be informed and trained. This concerns both breeders and veterinarians.

The means used to disseminate information are varied, with the authorities generally supplying brochures and posters, organizing training courses run by professional organizations, the relevant authorities or in collaboration with international bodies (FAO-WHO) and the media. To pass on the latest information quickly and in a targeted manner, some institutions will set up their own information dissemination system, such as a newsletter, website, news articles that will deal each time with new information or updates available (Diricks 2018).

III. Means of prevention

It's all about identifying problems before they emerge, through better prevention. At the same time, we need to be ready to manage epidemics and crises. We need to be more proactive than reactive in the face of emerging animal diseases. Not only does crisis management cost more than prevention, but, as already mentioned, crises can also undermine consumer confidence and public health. What's more, measures to combat animal diseases do not always result in their complete disappearance. Epidemics have consequences for farmers, society and the economy. The aim is therefore to prevent the emergence of these diseases or minimize their impact (Diricks 2018). The effectiveness of prevention and control policies relies on good governance and the quality of Veterinary Services, compliance with which with WHOA standards and guidelines on animal disease control is an indispensable prerequisite (OIE 2015).

1. Application of biosafety measures

1.1. General biosafety measures

All those involved in animal health must work together to constantly improve preventive measures. General biosecurity measures are :

* Compliance with good hygiene and husbandry practices on the farm.

*Animal identification and traceability;

* Monitoring imports at borders and illegal trade;

* Animal disease surveillance; (Diricks 2018).

To limit the risk of disease introduction from a given farm, the breeder must apply the following measures in collaboration with and under the supervision of the veterinary practitioner:

- <u>Introducing new animals to the farm :</u>

-Only buy animals with a health status equal to or better than that of the farm;

- Avoid animals that have passed through a market or assembly center, as they have been in contact with other animals and are at greater risk of introducing pathogens;

- Prevent sick animals from entering the farm;

- Isolate newly-introduced animals (quarantine) until the farm veterinarian's visit has taken place and/or the results of purchase tests are known;

- Minimize the introduction of animals from different origins into the farm, to limit the risk of introducing a sick animal;

- Comply with legislation on animal transport and trade (health certificates, hygiene, quarantine, etc.).

- Animal treatment :

- Isolate sick animals to monitor them and prevent transmission of the disease to other animals on the farm;

- Ensure adequate animal welfare. Animals housed in poorly ventilated barns or stressed animals are more susceptible to disease;

- Use appropriate, high-quality food.

- Avoid feeding kitchen waste, respect the target animal species and keep feeders clean;

- Care and treat animals properly, even for relatively innocent infections such as worms, mange, mites, etc., as these make them more vulnerable to other diseases;

- Apply the vaccination schedule as prescribed by the authorities

Visitors who come into professional contact with animals from other farms (veterinarians, technicians, inseminators, etc.) present a greater risk of introducing pathogens into a farm, which is why it is so important to manage access to the farm and prohibit it in certain situations.

- Visitor access to the farm :

- Use clothing belonging to the farm;

-Install foot baths to disinfect shoes at the entrance to stables;

- Observe hand hygiene;

- Keep unauthorized persons out of the barns by locking them, if possible;

- Keeping a logbook noting all visitors to the farm (name, date, reason for visit) is important in the event of an outbreak;

- Clean and disinfect equipment, vehicles and premises regularly (after each use) using approved disinfectants;

- Controlling pests and animals not belonging to the farm:

- Controlling pests such as rodents and insects, which can transmit disease,

- Prohibit pets such as dogs and cats from entering stables, etc. ;

- Prevent domestic animals from coming into contact with wild animals;

- Minimize contact between animals of different species;

- Properly manage carcasses by preventing access to other animals on the farm, storing them in a place that is easy to disinfect, removing them frequently, etc. ;

- When possible, use the "all in - all out" system and apply a sanitary vacuum (Diricks 2018).

1.2. Specific measures following detection of an emerging disease

Early detection is the key to rapid diagnosis and response, and to effective management of emerging animal diseases. Some emerging animal diseases are contagious, spreading rapidly and regardless of borders. Rapid response and management of animal disease at an early stage are essential for the implementation of effective biosecurity measures, the objectives of which are :

- Limit the spread of the disease to other farms and prevent an epidemic, or limit its consequences;

- Implement appropriate control measures and communicate them effectively;

- Reduce the cost, difficulty and scale of the fight and achieve better results.

The consequences of a disease or epidemic can be reduced if hazards are detected early and information is rapidly exchanged between the partners involved. A well-functioning network of breeders, veterinarians and authorities in the field, with optimal transmission of information, is of crucial importance in the fight against emerging animal diseases (Barnouin and VOURC'H 2004).

Biosecurity measures can be applied at several levels: at farm level, and during animal transport and trade, at the level of animal monitoring and early detection of animal diseases on the farm.

1.2.1. Measures applied by the breeder

Farmers are the first people who can prevent or limit the risk of introducing animal diseases into their farms. They can also prevent the spread of disease to other farms. By applying biosecurity measures, in collaboration with the veterinarian.

Farmers are the only ones who can observe and inspect the animals on their farm on a daily basis, detect any unusual signs or abnormal behavior in these animals, and contact the veterinarian as soon as possible. The veterinarian will assess the situation, decide what action to take if necessary (laboratory tests, reporting to the authorities, etc.) and, with the collaboration of the farmers, implement any necessary control measures.

1.2.2. Measures applied by the veterinary practitioner

Veterinary practitioners also have a vital role to play in ensuring optimal biosecurity to prevent the spread of pathogens, and in advising farmers on the best practices to implement.

Veterinary practitioners have a major responsibility in preventing and/or limiting the transmission of contagious diseases between farms. Veterinary practitioners are the right people to provide farmers with biosecurity advice to prevent the introduction of pathogens into farms.

Veterinary practitioners must avoid transporting pathogens between different farms or animals. The veterinary practitioner is therefore required to apply certain specific biosafety measures:

• Wash hands with disinfectant before and after each visit, and between handling different animals or animals from different batches;

• Use foot baths at the entrance and exit of each barn;

• Use the farm's own animal restraint equipment, or wash and disinfect restraint equipment between uses; this also applies to diagnostic equipment;

• Use a new needle for each animal, even if they come from the same farm or batch;

• Cars can be mechanical vectors of certain pathogens; we recommend parking them in a special area, as far away from the stables as possible, or preferably outside the farm;

• Wear farm shoes and clothing or disposable aprons (Diricks 2019).

Mandatory reporting is a very important concept. It is through mandatory reporting that the authorities have a chance of containing an epidemic of a contagious disease in time, i.e. before it reaches uncontrollable proportions.

1.1.3. Measures applied at country level

1.1.3.1. In wealthy countries

In high-income countries, the trend is to control the main infectious diseases by organizing surveillance (networks, plans, prophylaxis), controlling domestic animal movements, vaccinating or implementing other measures decided on a case-by-case basis (e.g. poultry confinement during migration periods to limit the risk of contamination by Influenza viruses). This risk control relies on the ability of stakeholders to finance animal health activities and the loss of income for producers (loss of income for breeders, trade restrictions, etc.) (Ministry of Agriculture 2023).

1.1.3.2. In developing countries

Low- and middle-income countries are generally more vulnerable, as they have less capacity to monitor animal diseases and implement animal health operations to deal with them. However, more than national income levels alone, it is above all the characteristics of the local food system (particularly in terms of animal population density) that condition the consequences of global warming (intensity and nature of effects) (Leboucq 2019). In regions with intensive, large-scale livestock farming, an epizootic can take on a wide scope and cause considerable macroeconomic impacts: epizootic outbreaks are favored by the concentration of individuals, and management includes restrictive measures (movement bans sometimes accompanied by the downgrading of health status in the sense of the World Organization for Animal Health (OIE), slaughter. The entire agricultural and commercial sector may be affected. In regions where family subsistence farming predominates, diseases often persist in an endemic form that can lead to crises. Only infected farms are then impacted (illness or death of animals leading to economic losses) (Ministry of Agriculture 2023).

2. Medical prophylaxis measures

2.1. Vaccination

Vaccination is very useful in the prevention and control of many diseases, as long as it is carried out in accordance with a health control program in force. However, vaccination alone will not achieve the desired results if the vaccination program is not integrated into an integrated control strategy based on a combination of control measures.

2.2. Vaccination strategy

If vaccination is one of the solutions chosen to prevent a disease, the country will ensure that the preconditions are met before launching a specific vaccination policy, to give it every chance of success.

Before implementation, it is essential to guarantee the quality of vaccines and define the conditions under which any vaccination policy will one day be discontinued (exit strategy).

2.3. Vaccines :

Vaccines must be manufactured in accordance with the international guidelines described in the WHO Manual of Diagnostic Tests and Vaccines for Terrestrial Animals. For most vaccines, the successful implementation of a vaccination campaign requires permanent respect of the cold chain (continuous temperature control). In some developing regions, WHOA has set up regional vaccine banks to support its member countries against rabies, foot-and-mouth disease and peste des petits ruminants in emergency situations (OIE 2015, WHOA 2024).

IV. The importance of communication

Communication is one of the most important tools in the fight against emerging diseases, for two reasons. Firstly, because the strict application of preventive measures conveyed by communication is the best tool for curbing any emerging disease , secondly, because in the case of known emerging diseases, healthcare teams have frequently come up against the incredulity, or even hostility, of the population (Seytre 2016). Emerging diseases are a highly publicized topic, highlighting the role played by research organizations in better understanding and controlling them. During each health crisis, researchers are much in demand, as in winter and spring 2006 with HPAI (interviews, articles and reports in the press, radio and TV). Scientific journals are very interested in information from fields at the heart of epidemiological cycles. It has thus been possible to publish results on HPAI, RVF and FWN in leading scientific journals (Camus and Lancelot 2007).

Collaboration and communication. If control measures still need to be implemented because the disease has nevertheless managed to establish itself and spread, collaboration and communication between all the partners involved is essential to the success of these control measures. The collaboration of farmers is also important in the context of visits by the farm veterinarian responsible for epidemiological surveillance of animal diseases

(Diricks 2018).

Rumors, misconceptions and hostility have, of course, sometimes deep cultural, social and political roots, which it would be illusory to hope to sweep away with a good communication strategy. But communication should, at the very least, make them recede rather than reinforce them (Seytre 2016).

1. Message development :

The development of risk communication messages needs to include building blocks such as technical information - the factual data and figures that support key messages; the cultural values of populations need to be taken into account; the individuals and Veterinary Services communicating about risk need to inspire trust (this is by far the most important factor!); the credibility of the spokesperson and the Veterinary Services; the expression of support and empathy.); credibility of the spokesperson and Veterinary Services; expression of support and empathy: people listen more willingly and are attentive to the message if they feel that the person communicating it is empathetic and concerned (WHOA 2015).

A message that follows good practice in animal health communication as presented in the WHOA guide is based on seven key terms, referred to as the 7 Cs (WHOA 2015):

Focusing attention; a message needs to polarize attention by getting to the point quickly and presenting convincing arguments.

Clarify messages: it's essential to clarify the meaning of the message, to explain the meaning of statistics and to explain the terminology used.

Communicate the benefits: you need to be explicit about the benefits, for example: "your cows will be healthier and produce more milk; this will protect your herd and consolidate your farm's income".

Rely on consistency: All data communicated must be consistent, including statistical and factual data, and calls for mobilization.

Consider the HEART and the HEAD: People perceive information communicated not only visually and aurally, but also through their feelings. Themes and messages that appeal to feelings and emotions are therefore more likely to be heard, understood and reacted to, opening the door to action and change.

Building trust: trust is built on the quality of the technical content, respect for the public's values, the credibility of the Veterinary Services or its speakers, and the interest they show.

Channeling towards action: In order to induce the desired change in behavior, communication MUST be channeled towards a watchword.

2. Messages to avoid:
Mistakes to avoid in communication are :

Messages with technical information only :

There is a widespread misconception among specialists that transparency and precision are the key to good risk communication. However, technical information (figures and factual data to support key messages), although central to risk communication, is far from sufficient. A message needs to be clear and adapted to the target population.

Messages prohibiting daily or traditional activities: messages promoting behavioural change

A systematic communication error stemming from the undifferentiated communication strategy, which consists in calling for changes in behavior when the emerging disease is not a concrete threat. In the "pre-epidemic period", the WHO recommends disseminating "key messages to reduce risk behaviors and facilitate the adoption of practices that prevent infection or reduce community transmission". Otherwise, these messages will be confronted with a certainty reinforced by daily experience, since despite everything the population hears, they will continue their activities without the disease appearing. As Wilkinson and Leach point out, "erroneous awareness that conflicts with people's experience creates mistrust". This kind of message must be avoided, as it has no effectiveness in preventing emerging disease and combating an ongoing epidemic; not only does it dilute the essential messages, generating a useless waste of energy, but above all it discredits all communication on the disease in question, in a context where disbelief is a major obstacle to successful prevention (Wilkinson and Leach 2015, Seytre 2016).

Unscientific or harmful messages:

These messages dilute communication on the real precautions to be taken, but they can only increase mistrust. What is the public to think when faced with an accumulation of recommendations and messages that are unrelated, disproved by experience and, of course, unsupported by any explanation?

It has long been demonstrated that coercion alone is ineffective in the fight against an emerging disease, which can only rely on the trust and support of populations (Seytre 2016).

Anxiety-provoking messages:

A strategic error in communication about an emerging disease is that it is not modulated according to the risk actually incurred, disseminating messages in disease-free countries that should only target epidemic areas. the WHO recommends "in the pre-epidemic period" to "disseminate simplified case definitions" for "community-based surveillance" (Seytre 2016).

3. Communicating messages :

Messages can be communicated in three main ways:

- By drafting and distributing simple, complete and explicit reports, usually reserved for the authorities, to explain the situation.

• Through meetings and discussions, mainly with various partners (ministries) and the scientific community.

• Through local, regional and national media, mainly to present the situation to the general public.

• Posters, flyers, etc.: a widely used method for disseminating information and warnings in administrations, schools, airports...

The Veterinary Services spokesperson is the person most in demand during disease outbreaks, and their role is to communicate the information the audience wants or needs, in order to prevent and reduce hazards, disease spread and animal mortality. The spokesperson can breathe life into the Services, building a foundation of trust and credibility, and gathering support for the animal health and welfare response. Veterinary Services will often be asked to speak out on emerging and zoonotic diseases (WHOA 2015).

Conclusion

Climate change and environmental change are just part of the range of changes affecting ecosystems and favoring the emergence and re-emergence of animal diseases. Infectious diseases that were thought to have been conquered at the end of the 20th century are back in the spotlight as new ones emerge or re-emerge. More often than not, the cause of changes in the epidemiological situation is not unique, but multifactorial; however, it is important to be aware of the importance of human factors in these developments. The complex interactions of climate change with hosts, vectors and the environment have facilitated the spread of a number of viruses, including bluetongue in Europe, Rift Valley fever in Africa and highly virulent influenza viruses in Asia.

In order to combat these emerging or re-emerging diseases effectively, it is essential to detect them as early as possible. Early detection and rapid diagnosis of emerging animal diseases are vital for rapid response, effective action and damage limitation in the event of an epidemic. In this context, epidemiological surveillance and investigation play a vital role. In addition, as many of these diseases are zoonoses, a balanced collaboration between doctors and veterinarians, in line with that advocated by the "one health" concept, seems essential for better monitoring of emergencies (Dufour 2017).

References

1. Afssa (2005). Rapport sur l'évaluation du risque d'apparition et de développement de maladies animales compte tenu d'un éventuel réchauffement climatique.
2. Ajana, F. and e. al (2022). ePILLY Trop tropical infectious diseases
3. Akther, M., S. H. Akter, S. Sarker, J. W. Aleri, H. Annandale, S. Abraham and J. M. Uddin (2023). "Global burden of lumpy skin disease, outbreaks, and future challenges." Viruses **15**(9): 1861.
4. Angot, J.-L. (2009). "Surveillance and control of import risks of infectious animal diseases: the role of the OIE and veterinary services." Bulletin de l'Académie nationale de médecine **193**(8): 1861-1870.
5. Badillo, A. (2024, 12-03-2024). "Global warming: causes and consequences" Retrieved 28-9-2024, 2024, from https://climate.selectra.com/fr/comprendre/rechauffement- climate.
6. Barnouin, J. and I. Sache (2010). Les maladies émergentes: épidémiologie chez le végétal, l'animal et l'homme, Éditions Quae.
7. Barnouin, J. and G. VOURC'H (2004). "Emerging diseases: a challenge for the sustainable development of animal production." INRAE Productions Animales **17**(5): 355-363.
8. Ben Ali, M. and a. al (2022). "Serological survey of rift valley fever in camelids in Tunisia." Bulletin zoosanitaire **24**: 10-15.
9. Black, P. and M. Nunn (2009). Impact of climate and environmental change on emerging and re-emerging animal diseases on livestock production Climate change has a significant impact on the emergence and re-emergence of animal diseases. OIE. Paris **1-13**.
10. Bouaicha, F., A. Eisenbarth, K. Elati, A. Schulz, B. B. Smida, M. Bouajila, L. Sassi, M. Rekik, M. H. Groschup and M. K. Khbou (2021). "Epidemiological investigation of Crimean-Congo haemorrhagic fever virus infection among the one-humped camels (Camelus dromedarius) in southern Tunisia." Ticks and tick-borne diseases **12**(1): 101601.
11. Bouchard, C., A. Dibernardo, J. Koffi, H. Wood, P. Leighton and L. Lindsay (2019). "Increased risk of tick-borne diseases in the context of climate and environmental change." Canada Communicable Disease Report **45**: 89-98.
12. Brugère-Picoux, J. and B. Chomel (2009). "Risks of introduction and establishment in Europe of exotic infectious diseases." Bulletin de l'Académie nationale de médecine **193**(8): 1805-1819.
13. Camus, E. and R. Lancelot (2007). "Emerging animal diseases: challenges and opportunities." Bulletin de l'Académie vétérinaire de France **160**(3): 223-228.
14. Carlson, C. J., G. F. Albery, C. Merow, C. H. Trisos, C. M. Zipfel, E. A. Eskew, K. J. Olival, N. Ross and S. Bansal (2022). "Climate change increases cross-species viral transmission risk." Nature **607**(7919): 555-562.
15. Cheung, W. W., J. L. Sarmiento, J. Dunne, T. L. Frolicher, V. *W.* Lam, M. Deng Palomares, R. Watson and D. Pauly (2013). "Shrinking of fishes exacerbates

impacts of global ocean changes on marine ecosystems." Nature Climate Change **3**(3): 254-258.

16. Chevalier, V., F. Courtin, H. Guis, A. Tran and L. Vial (2015). "Climate change and vector-borne Animal diseases." Climate Change and World Agricultures: 96.
17. Choumet, V. (2021). "Coping with the emergence of infectious viral diseases, a contemporary challenge." Actualités Pharmaceutiques **60**(608): 16-20.
18. Das, M., M. S. R. Chowdhury, S. Akter, A. K. Mondal, M. J. Uddin, M. M. Rahman and M. M. Rahman (2021). "An updated review on lumpy skin disease: perspective of Southeast Asian countries." J. adv. biotechnol. exp. ther **4**(3): 322-333.
19. Diricks, H. (2018). Emerging animal diseases A. F. p. l. S. d. l. C. Food.
20. Diricks, H. (2019). Emerging animal diseases.
21. Information brochure for veterinarians. A. F. p. l. S. d. l. C. Food.
22. Dufour, B. (2017). "The causes of the emergence of infectious diseases." Bulletin de l'Académie Nationale de Médecine **201**(7-9): 1189-1195.
23. Dungu, B. and A. Anyamba (2020). "Rift Valley fever: a recurrent health emergency that needs to be organized against." WHOA Bulletin: 6.
24. FAO (2020). Animal health and climate change, Food and Agriculture Organization of the United Nations
25. Gérin, M., P. Gosselin, S. Cordier, C. Viau, P. Quénel and É. Dewailly (2003). Environnement et santé publique: Fondements et pratiques, Édisem/Tec & Doc.
26. Githeko, A. K., S. W. Lindsay, U. E. Confalonieri and J. A. Patz (2001). "Climate change and vector-borne diseases: a regional analysis." Bulletin of the World Health Organization: the international journal of public health: collection of articles 2001; 4: 6272.
27. Hassine, T. B., J. Amdouni, F. Monaco, G. Savini, S. Sghaier, I. B. Selimen, *W.* Chandoul, K. B. Hamida and S. Hammami (2017). "Emerging vector-borne diseases in dromedaries in Tunisia: West Nile, bluetongue, epizootic haemorrhagic disease and Rift Valley fever." Onderstepoort Journal of Veterinary Research **84**(1): 1-3.
28. Huntington, B., T. M. Bernardo, M. Bondad-Reantaso, M. Bruce, B. Devleesschauwer, W. Gilbert, D. Grace, A. Havelaar, M. Herrero and T. L. Marsh (2021). "Global Burden of Animal Diseases: a novel approach to understanding and managing disease in livestock and aquaculture." OIE Scientific and Technical Review **40**(2): 567-584.
29. Jansen, A., E. Luge, B. Guerra, P. Wittschen, A. D. Gruber, C. Loddenkemper, T. Schneider, M. Lierz, D. Ehlert and B. Appel (2007). "Leptospirosis in urban wild boars, Berlin, Germany." Emerging infectious diseases **13**(5): 739.
30. Khamassi Khbou, M., R. Romdhane, F. Bouaicha Zaafouri, M. Bouajila, L. Sassi, S. K. Appelberg, A. Schulz, A. Mirazimi, M. H. Groschup and M. Rekik (2021). "Presence of antibodies to Crimean Congo haemorrhagic fever virus in sheep in Tunisia, North Africa." Veterinary medicine and science **7**(6): 2323-2329.

31. Leboucq, N. (2019). "Issues related to high-burden endemic diseases in the south." Bulletin de l'Académie Vétérinaire de France **172**(1): 22-27.
32. Ludwig, A., H. Zheng, L. Vrbova, M. Drebot, M. Iranpour and L. Lindsay (2019). "Increased risk of endemic mosquito-borne diseases in Canada due to climate change." Canada Communicable Disease Report **45**(4): 99-107.
33. Masson-Delmotte, V., P. Zhai, A. Pirani, S. Connors, C. Péan, S. Berger and B. Zhouj (2021). Climate Change 2021. The physical scientific basis, Cambridge, Cambridge University Press.
34. MelloukiHanane (2023). Contribution à l'analyse du régime climatique de quelques stations de l'Est algérien, university center of abdalhafid boussouf-MILA.
35. Miner, K. R., M. R. Turetsky, E. Malina, A. Bartsch, J. Tamminen, A. D. McGuire, A. Fix, C. Sweeney, C. D. Elder and C. E. Miller (2022). "Permafrost carbon emissions in a changing Arctic." Nature Reviews Earth & Environment **3**(1): 55-67.
36. Ministry of Agriculture, d. l. s. a. e. d. l. f. (2023). "Animal disease control in the context of climate change - Analysis No. 184." Retrieved 27-9-2024, 2024, from https://agriculture.gouv.fr/la-lutte-contre-les-maladies-animales-dans-le-contexte-du- changement-climatique.
37. NationsUnies. (2018, 9-3-2018). "Animal disease control: more than 4,700 veterinarians trained in 25 countries by FAO and USAID." Health Retrieved 1-10-2024, 2024.
38. United Nations. (2024). "Climate Action" Climate Change Retrieved 27-9-2024, 2024, from https://www.un.org/fr/climatechange/what-is-climate-change.
39. Ng, V., E. Rees, L. Lindsay, M. Drebot, T. Brownstone, T. Sadeghieh and S. Khan (2019). "Could climate change lead to the spread of exotic mosquito-borne diseases in Canada." Canada Communicable Disease Report **45**(4): 108-118.
40. Noël, H. and S. publique France (2019). Climate change and infectious risk: known, unknown and unrecognized impacts. 20th Journées Internationales D'Infectiologie Lyon - France.
41. Ogden, N. and P. Gachon (2019). "Climate change and infectious diseases: What can we expect." Canada Communicable Disease Report **45**(4): 83-88.
42. OIE (2015). Prevention and control of animal diseases. WHOA. Online version: www.oie.int
43. Olivero, J., J. E. Fa, M. Á. Farfán, A. L. Márquez, R. Real, F. J. Juste, S. A. Leendertz and R. Nasi (2020). "Human activities link fruit bat presence to Ebola virus disease outbreaks." Mammal Review **50**(1): 1-10.
44. WHO. (2024). "Emerging diseases." Health Topics Retrieved 27-9-2024, 2024, from **https://www.emro.who.int/fr/health-topics/emerging-diseases/Page-1.html.**
45. WHOA (2015). Communication guide for veterinary services
46. WHOA. (2024). "Who are we?" Retrieved 3-10-2024, from https://www.woah.org/fr/qui-nous-sommes/.
47. Pepin, M., P. Boireau, F. Boué, J. Castric, F. Cliquet, Y. Douzal, A. Jestin, F.

Moutou and S. Zientara (2007). "Emergence of animal and human infectious diseases." INRAE Productions Animales **20**(3): 199-206.
48. Perrin, L., G. Limon-Vega and S. Bacigalupo (2024). Lumpy Skin Disease in North Africa, Department for Environment, Food and Rural Affairs
49. Puget, J.-L., R. Blanchet, J. Salençon and A. Carpentier (2010). le changement climatique, Institut de France- Académie des sciences**:** 24.
50. Quiggin, D., K. De Meyer, L. Hubble-Rose and A. Froggatt (2021). Climate change risk assessment 2021
51. Rekik, S., I. Hammami, O. Timoumi, D. Maghzaoua, M. Khamassi Khbou, A. Schulz, M. H. Groschup and M. Gharbi (2024). "A Review on Crimean-Congo Hemorrhagic Fever Infections in Tunisia." Vector-Borne and Zoonotic Diseases.
52. Sanguine, Y. (2021). One health Emerging animal diseases under surveillance. Dossier de presse CIRAD**:** 32.
53. Seguin, B. and J.-F. Soussana (2008). "Greenhouse gas emissions and climate change: causes and observed consequences for agriculture and livestock." Le Courrier de l'environnement de l'INRA **55**(55): 79-91.
54. Selmi, R., A. Mamlouk, M. B. Said, H. B. Yahia, H. Abdelaali, F. B. Chehida, M. Daaloul-Jedidi, A. Gritli and L. Messadi (2020). "First serological evidence of the Rift Valley fever Phlebovirus in Tunisian camels." Acta tropica **207**: 105462.
55. Seytre, B. (2016). "The wanderings of Ebola virus disease communication." Bull Soc Pathol Exot **109**(4): 314-323.
56. Shongo, M. Y. P., T. K. Lubala, O. Mukuku, A. K. Mutombo, P. M. Bunga, A. M. Tambwe, M. B. Ekwalanga, O. N. Luboya and S. O. Wembonyama (2020). "Emerging infectious diseases: transmission and epidemiology." PAMJ-One Health **3**(11).
57. Swynghedauw, B. and J.-L. Wemeau (2021). "Report 20-07. Consequences of climate change on human and animal health." Bulletin de l'Académie Nationale de Médecine **205**(3): 219-226.
58. Tazerji, S. S., R. Nardini, M. Safdar, A. A. Shehata and P. M. Duarte (2022). "An overview of anthropogenic actions as drivers for emerging and re-emerging zoonotic diseases." Pathogens **11**(11): 1376.
59. Thornton, P. K., P. G. Jones, G. Alagarswamy, J. Andresen and M. Herrero (2010). "Adapting to climate change: agricultural system and household impacts in East Africa." Agricultural systems **103**(2): 73-82.
60. Toma, B. and E. Thiry (2003). "What is an emerging disease." Epidemiology and Animal Health **44**: 1-11.
61. Tuppurainen, E. and N. Galon (2016). Lumpy skin disease: Current situation in Europe and neighbouring regions and Control measures needed to stop its spread in south-eastern Europe OIE European Regional Commission**:** 12.
62. Valingot, M., M. Chaumien, C. Sourd and P. Cannet (2015). Impacts of climate change on species WWF**:** 21.
63. Wang, W.-H., A. Thitithanyanont, A. N. Urbina and S.-F. Wang (2021). Emerging and re-emerging diseases, MDPI. **10:** 827.
64. Wannous, C. (2024). The importance of the "One Health" approach to combat

emerging and re-emerging zoonotic epidemics and pandemics-The animal health perspective. General D. d. p., World Organization for Animal Health.
65. Wilkinson, A. and M. Leach (2015). "Briefing: Ebola-myths, realities, and structural violence." African Affairs **114**(454): 136-148.
66. Wright, P. F. (2022). "Infectious diseases in animals: the importance of diagnosis."
67. Zouaghi, K., A. Bouattour, H. Aounallah, R. Surtees, E. Krause, J. Michel, A. Mamlouk, A. Nitsche and Y. M'ghirbi (2021). "First serological evidence of Crimean-Congo hemorrhagic fever virus and Rift Valley fever virus in ruminants in Tunisia." Pathogens **10**(6): 769.

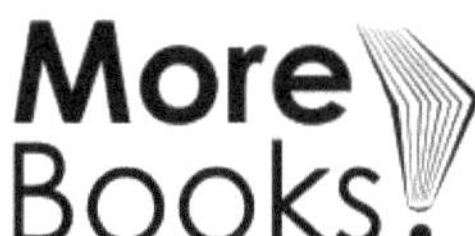
More
Books!

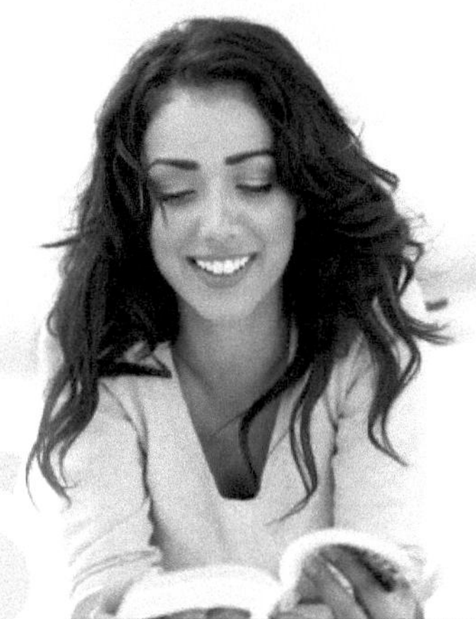

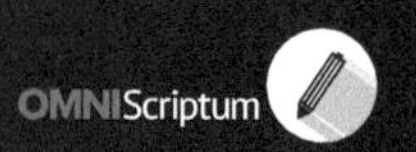
OMNIScriptum

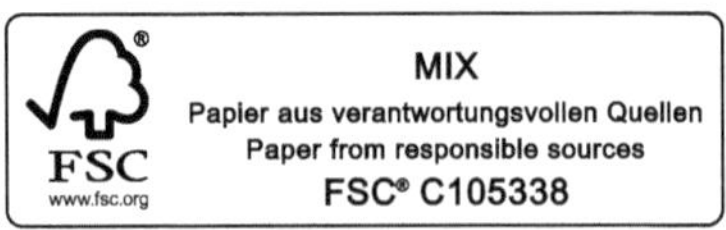

Printed by Books on Demand GmbH, Norderstedt / Germany